MW01048055

24-Week Health Plan

By Karen Breitbart

Published by Totline
an imprint of
Frank Schaffer Publications®

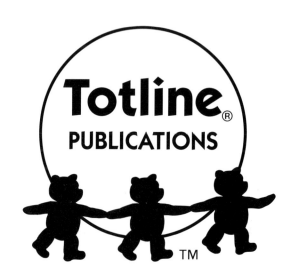

Author: Karen Breitbart
Editor: Mary Hassinger

Frank Schaffer Publications®

Totline Publications is an imprint of Frank Schaffer Publications.

Send all inquiries to:
Frank Schaffer Publications
3195 Wilson Drive NW
Grand Rapids, Michigan 49534

24-Week Health Plan

ISBN 1-57029-549-2

1 2 3 4 5 6 7 8 9 MAZ 11 10 09 08 07 06

Table of Contents

Introduction

American society has acknowledged obesity as a growing concern. While we want our children to be healthy, active, and happy, safety concerns have kept children indoors, using television shows, computers, and video games to fill hours that used to be spent playing kickball, football, skating, and running around local neighborhoods. Even bike riding has become hazardous with the increase in traffic patterns.

Obesity in children has been noted in classrooms across our nation. Obese children do not choose free-running play times in school, preferring more sedate forms of exercise. Aggravating the lack of exercise is the lure of convenient fast food restaurants offering children kid's meals that contain various bonus games and toys. When we combine these two things with children's natural tendency towards being "picky eaters" it is no wonder that we have a national concern on our hands.

Children do not need to diet though. What they do need is adequate food for proper growth, which does not contain an overabundant amount of sugar and saturated fats. Children need education on how to identify and choose healthy foods.

Most children have definite food likes and dislikes. Dietitians and nutritionists recommend that parents make a wide variety of foods available to children. They also suggest encouraging children to taste and experience new foods in small quantities, without forcing the issue. When a variety of food is available, and unnecessary pressure does not make trying new food a "battle of wills," children often accept and enjoy new foods. Nutrition experts suggest that children should not be told to "clean their plates," and children should be allowed to choose their portion sizes. Experts also suggest repeat tasting of foods that children have not enjoyed in the past. The *rule of seven* proposes that it is sometimes necessary to taste a new food seven times before a taste for this food is developed. The *rule of seven* advises "tasting" be separated by several days. Children may enjoy keeping track of the number of times they have tasted a new food. It is also beneficial for parents to remind children of other new foods that they have *learned* to enjoy. (After all, don't most babies reject ice cream the first time they try it because of the different temperature and texture?) Nutritionists point out that children who watch their parents enjoy a variety of foods are more likely to have an open mind when it comes to trying new foods.

Other health professionals emphasize the importance of establishing healthful nutrition attitudes and practices during the early childhood years. It is well documented that diet and exercise patterns developed during these years set the stage for life-long habits. The ultimate goal of nutrition education for preschool-age children is that they learn that a well-balanced diet contains a wide variety of foods. When it comes to providing their children with good nutrition, parents clearly face a daunting but essential task. Because of the long-term health effects of poor childhood diets and the many diseases that are known to have a dietary component, the stakes are high.

In addition to healthy eating, most people will agree that there are many benefits to physical activity and exercise as well. We know that leading an active lifestyle can help develop strong muscles and bones, increase flexibility, and can help people maintain a healthy weight.

Most people also will agree that our nation, as a whole, does not get enough physical activity or exercise. This is evidenced by the rise in obesity seen all around America. Sadly, this also can be seen in our classrooms.

Several factors have been identified as contributing to this condition. First is the rise in popularity of video games, as well as the continuing proliferation of computers and televisions in our homes (and even in children's rooms), lead to many children having a lot of "down time." In addition, many parents are hesitant to let their children play outside, unless they are within narrow and supervised boundaries. The result of this is that children are spending less time building healthy bodies through active play and more time playing in sedentary positions.

But, it doesn't have to be that way forever. Children can achieve many physical and emotional benefits from physical activity. Regular physical activity can help relieve anxiety and stress, increase self-esteem, and reduce the risk of type-2 diabetes. It has been found that participating in regular physical activities can also help children develop social skills such as sharing, turn taking, and cooperation. Exercise also helps children develop physical skills, coordination, flexibility, and balance. Exercising with others, whether in a casual or organized setting helps children develop a sense of belonging. Children who have time to "play hard" and be "physical" are able to concentrate for longer periods of time. Recent studies show that children who exercise regularly score higher on standardized tests. Introducing and encouraging an active lifestyle will not only increase a child's physical and mental well being, but also it may help them avoid later health problems.

There are many ways to encourage children to enjoy physical activities. Many suggested activities are ones which children naturally enjoy. Activities such as walking, running, skipping, and riding a bicycle or scooter will benefit a child's physical being. Kicking, throwing, catching, and bouncing balls will not only help keep a child active, but also will develop hand-eye coordination. Playing in playgrounds is a good way for children to develop strong hearts and bodies. Swimming also provides many physical benefits for children, but it must be supervised. Dancing, gymnastics, and martial arts (at a non-competitive level) also can benefit a child's physical and mental health. Playing or walking a family (or a neighbor's) pet can keep a child active and also can build a child's sense of responsibility and self-esteem. Organized sports programs help children develop skills that can be enjoyed throughout their lives.

Physical activity and exercise should also be encouraged in school. This book contains activities that can help lead children to a healthy lifestyle. Movement and exercise activities are provided and will help the children develop coordination and gross-motor abilities while strengthening cardio-vascular health. Stretching activities are important, too. They help develop good flexibility and decrease the chances of injury during sports or play. The games included are designed to give children an opportunity to practice physical skills and to assist children in developing cooperation and good

sportsmanship. Teachers and children will not only enjoy the physical activities, but they will also reap benefits such as increased health, concentration, balance, flexibility, coordination, and self-esteem.

The National Center for Disease Control (CDC) uses the Body Mass Index (BMI) to measure overweight and obesity in the general adult population. Calculating the BMI is one of the easiest and consistent methods for assessment of a person's weight. A person's BMI allows him or her to compare their own weight status to the general population. The only information needed to calculate a person's BMI is the person's height and weight. A BMI formula is used to convert this information to a BMI. *The 24-Week Health Plan* contains BMI charts for girls and boys, along with instructions for finding and charting a person's BMI. This information can and should be shared with the parents.

The 24-Week Health Plan also contains lessons and activities that will help children learn about the benefits of healthy eating and daily physical activity. *The 24-Week Health Plan* provides a monthly letter to send home to the parents that will help keep them informed of the monthly health goals and lessons. The letter contains information as well as tips for incorporating the healthy food choices and physical activities taught at school.

Lessons are contained in *The 24-Week Health Plan* which introduce the children to the guidelines for healthy diets, set by United States Department of Agriculture (USDA). These engaging lessons will teach the children about the five food groups through hands-on activities, games, songs, and poems. These lessons will also teach and encourage the children to incorporate healthy food choices into their diets.

The 24-Week Health Plan is divided into six sections. The first section introduces the USDA's newest food pyramid, while the rest of the sections' focus on a specific food group. Also included, is a variety of recipes, containing main ingredients from each of the food groups. The children will receive numerous opportunities and encouragement to try new foods during the course of the six-month health plan.

In addition to encouraging healthy eating, *The 24-Week Health Plan* promotes an active lifestyle by introducing and encouraging the children to participate in a multitude of activities, exercises, and games. Stretching and yoga positions are also introduced. The children will be encouraged to utilize these physical skills and activities at home as well. Gross motor skills will be incorporated each month. A separate checklist is provided for keeping track of gross motor milestones for children ages three to six.

The 24-Week Health Plan will help any teacher, day care provider, or health professional plan and implement a program to teach about and promote healthy eating and exercise habits for young children

Complete Recommended Book List

Book Links for Month One

Eat Healthy, Feel Great by Martha Sears
(Little, Brown, 2002)

The Edible Pyramid: Good Eating Every Day
by Loreen Leedy (Holiday House, 1996)

Gregory, the Terrible Eater by Mitchell Sharmat
(Scholastic, 1985)

*Let's Exercise! (The Library of Healthy Living:
Staying Healthy)* by Alice B. McGinty
(Franklin Watts, 1999)

Milk: From Cow to Carton by Aliki
(HarperCollins Publishers, 1992)

The Milk Makers by Gail Gibbons
(Aladdin Library, 1987)

Stone Soup: An Old Tale by Marcia Brown
(Aladdin Picture Books, 1997)

The Very Hungry Caterpillar by Eric Carle
(Putnam Publishing Group, 1983

Book Links for Month Two

Bread and Jam For Frances by Russell and Lillian
Hoban (HarperTrophy, 1993)

Bread, Bread, Bread by Ann Morris
(HarperTrophy, 1993)

Bread is For Eating by David and Phyllis
Gershator (Henry Holt and Company, 1995)

Everyone Eats Bread by Janet Reed
(Yellow Umbrella Books, 2003)

Everybody Brings Noodles by Norah Dooley,
Peter J. Thornton (Carolrhoda Books, 1995)

The Little Red Hen by Paul Galdone
(Clarion Books, 1985)

The Little Red Hen (Makes a Pizza!)
by Philemon Sturges (Dutton Children's
Books, 1999)

Pancakes, Pancakes! by Eric Carle
(Scholastic Inc., New York, 1990)

The Tortilla Factory by Gary Paulsen, Ruth
Paulsen (Voyager Books, 1998)

Book Links for Month Three

Babar's Yoga for Elephants by Laurent De
Brunhoff (Harry N Abrams, 2002)

Eating the Alphabet by Lois Ehlert
(Red Wagon Books, 1996)

Exercise by Sharon Gordon
(Children's Press, 2002)

Gregory, the Terrible Eater by Mitchell Sharmat
(Scholastic, 1985)

Bunnies and Their Sports by Nancy L. Carlson
(Puffin Books, 1989)

Dog Food by Joost Elffers
(Arthur A. Levine Books, 2002)

Food For Thought by Joost Elffers
(Arthur A. Levine Books, 2005)

From Head to Toe by Eric Carle
(HarperCollins, 1997)

From Seed to Plant by Gail Gibbons
(Holiday House, 1993)

Growing Vegetable Soup by Lois Ehlert
(Voyager Books, 1990)

How Are You Peeling? by Joost Elffers
(Arthur A. Levine Books, 1999)

The Very Hungry Caterpillar by Eric Carle
(Putnam Publishing Group, 1983)

We're Going on a Bear Hunt by Michael Rosen
(Aladdin Library, 2003)

Book Links for Month Four
Apple Valley Year by Ann Turner
(Simon & Schuster Children's Publishing, 1993)

Eating the Alphabet by Lois Ehlert
(Red Wagon Books, 1996)

Dog Food by Joost Elffers
(Arthur A. Levine Books, 2002)

Food For Thought by Joost Elffers
(Arthur A. Levine Books, 2005)

From Blossom to Fruit (Apples)
by Gail Saunders-Smith (Capstone Press, 1997)

From Seed to Plant by Gail Gibbons
(Holiday House, 1993)

Growing Colors by Bruce McMillan
(HarperTrophy, 1994)

How Are You Peeling? by Joost Elffers (Arthur
A. Levine Books, 1999)

Book Links for Month Five
From Cow to Ice Cream by Bertram T. Knight
(Children's Press, 1997)

It Looked Like Spilt Milk by Charles G. Shaw
(HarperTrophy, 1988)

Milk and Cookies: A Frank Asch Bear Story
by Frank Asch (Parents Magazine Press, 1982)

Milk: From Cow to Carton by Aliki
(HarperTrophy, 1992)

Milk to Ice Cream by Inez Snyder
(Children's Press, 2003)

The Milk Makers by Gail Gibbons
(Aladdin Library, 1987)

Book Links for Month Six
A Passion for Proteins by Kristin Petrie
(Checkerboard Books, 2003)

Eat Healthy, Feel Great by Martha Sears
(Little, Brown, 2002)

The Edible Pyramid: Good Eating Every Day
by Loreen Leedy (Holiday House, 1996)

Meat and Protein by Robin Nelson
(Lerner Publications, 2003)

Meats and Protein by Jill Kalz (Smart Apple
Media, 2003)

Pyramid Pal — Meat, Poultry, Fish by Susan
Dawson (Griffin Publishing Group, 2000)

Web Links

http://www.mypyramid.gov

http://kidshealth.org

http://www.usda.gov

Comprehensive Materials List

The following are lists of materials that will come in handy as you work with your children for the next twenty-four weeks of this health plan. They are not arranged in any specific order, so read each month's plans before you begin, making sure that everything is ready.

For the recipes

- ☐ Measuring spoons
- ☐ Measuring cups
- ☐ Mixing bowls
- ☐ Mixing spoons
- ☐ Spatula
- ☐ Heat source
- ☐ Plastic tableware
- ☐ Paper cups
- ☐ Paper plates
- ☐ Napkins
- ☐ One sharp knife (adult use only)
- ☐ Anti-bacterial cleaner

As you go through the many healthy experiences in this plan keep several thoughts in mind:
- Food allergies
- Limits to physical activity for some children
- Family involvement is key
- Guest speakers or demonstrators are fun
- Use music as accompaniment to exercise

Miscellaneous supplies

- ☐ Poster board
- ☐ Chart paper
- ☐ Tape
- ☐ Glue
- ☐ Paint
- ☐ Paintbrushes
- ☐ Markers
- ☐ Crayons
- ☐ Pencils
- ☐ Newspaper
- ☐ Assortment of plastic and play food items
- ☐ Magazines
- ☐ Clean foam trays
- ☐ Empty boxes and containers from food items
- ☐ Cash register
- ☐ Grocery bags
- ☐ Play money
- ☐ Small food scale
- ☐ Orange cones
- ☐ Variety of balls
- ☐ Hula Hoops™
- ☐ Jump ropes

Published by Totline. Copyright protected. 1-57029-519-2 *24-Week Health Plan*

The USDA has released a new version of the traditional Food Pyramid—the visual that we have used for years to help make healthy food choices. This version provides many options to help guide us as we make food and activity choices every day.

The main messages about food choices come from the 2005 Dietary Guidelines for Americans. These messages focus on ideas such as making whole grains part of the grain group choices you make each day and choosing low-fat or fat-free dairy rather than whole milk and cheese. Information on the importance of eating the different types or "colors" of vegetables and how they each provide their own unique vitamins and minerals is included, as well as advice on how to eat the daily recommended amounts of each food group without feeling as though you are struggling to find options.

The importance of activity in a person's daily life is also a part of this new version of the Food Pyramid. Advice and pointer for adults as well as children are available on the main Web site for the Food Pyramid. This Web site is: http://www.mypyramid.gov

Pages 12–14 have visual resources for you to use as a guide with your children as you work on the 24-week health plan. Help the children to become familiar with the food groups and the many delicious choices that they have when getting their daily amounts of food and nutrition. Be sure to share this information with the families in your group. They will want to learn about making good choices for their children.

Use the Food Pyramid Mini-Poster on page 12 as the basis or focus of a small classroom display. Post it in the center of a bulletin board or poster board. Use the Food Pyramid Cards found on pages 13–14 to expand the display, explaining the different food groups and the different foods that belong to each group. Make the display even more meaningful to the children by having them cut pictures from magazines of food choices that they could make. Have them attach the items to the bulletin board under the appropriate Food Group Cards.

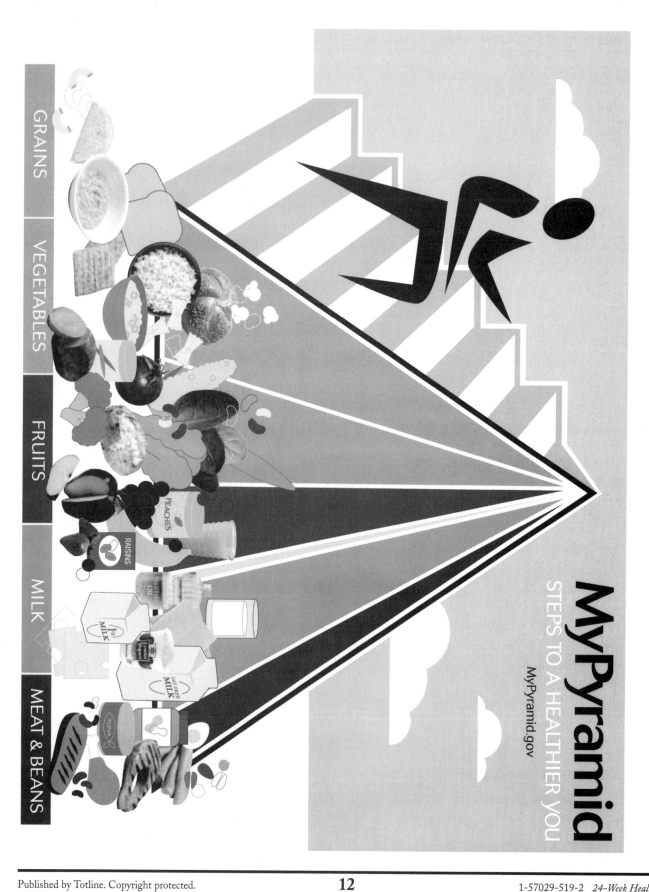

GRAINS

Eat 6 oz. every day: at least half should be whole grain

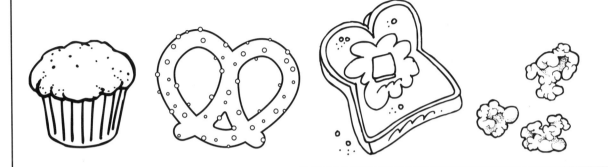

VEGETABLES

Eat 2 $\frac{1}{2}$ cups every day

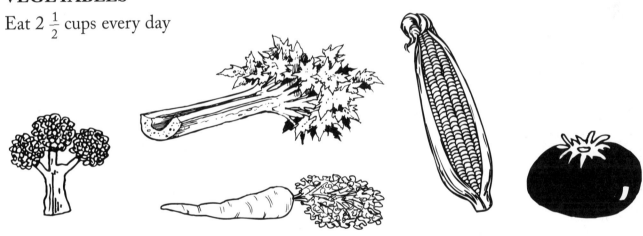

FRUITS

Eat 1 $\frac{1}{2}$ cups every day

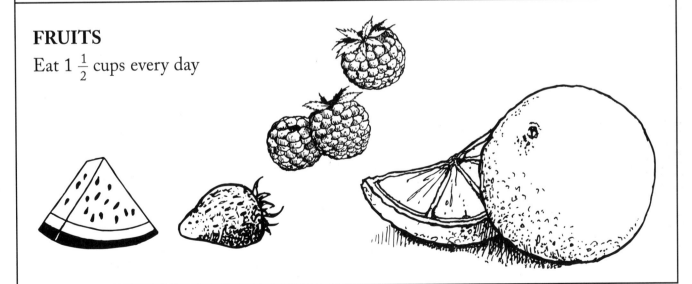

Food Pyramid Cards

MILK

Get 3 cups every day

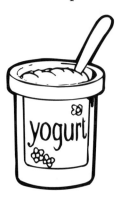
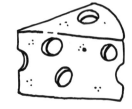
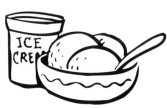
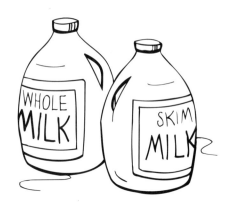

MEAT and BEANS

Eat 5 oz. every day

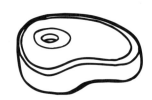
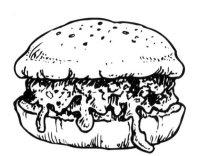
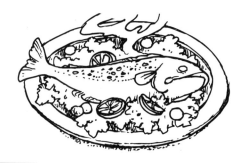
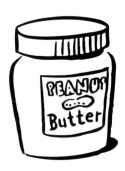

OILS/FATS and SUGARS

Not food groups on the Pyramid, but know your limits every day.

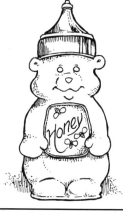
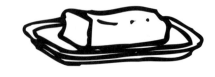

How Much Do We Need to Eat?

Food Group	Food Item	Normal Portion Size
GRAIN	Bread	
VEGETABLE	Carrots	
FRUITS	Apple	
MILK	Glass of milk	
MEAT AND BEANS	Piece of chicken	

1-57029-549-2 *24-Week Health Plan*

Children's Body Mass Index (BMI)

The National Center for Disease Control (CDC) uses the Body Mass Index (BMI) to measure overweight and obesity in the general adult population. Calculating the BMI is one of the easiest and consistent methods for assessment of a person's weight. A person's BMI allows him or her to compare their own weight status to the general population. The only information needed to calculate a person's BMI is the person's height and weight. A BMI formula is used to convert this information to a BMI.

How to calculate Body Mass Index Number (BMI):

1. Measure the child's height.

2. Weigh the child.

3. Use the following formula to find the child's BMI number:
   - Weight in pounds ÷ Height in Inches ÷ Height in Inches x 703 = BMI

4. Use the CDC BMI-for-age gender specific chart. Mark the intersection point of child's age and his/her BMI. Look at the series of curved lines where the point lies to determine his or her BMI number.

The following web site has a BMI calculator:

http://www.cdc.gov

Teachers: document each child's BMI on an individual chart (see pages 17–18) before starting the 24-Week Health Plan. It is also a good idea to share this information with the parents or caretakers of the students.

The CDC's National Center for Health Statistics established the following percentile cutoff points to identify underweight and overweight children:

Underweight	BMI-for-age: less than the 5th percentile
Normal Weight	BMI-for-age: from 5th percentile to less than the 85th percentile
At-Risk for Overweight	BMI-for-age: from 85th percentile to less than 95th percentile
Overweight	BMI-for-age: greater than 95th percentile

CDC Growth Charts: United States

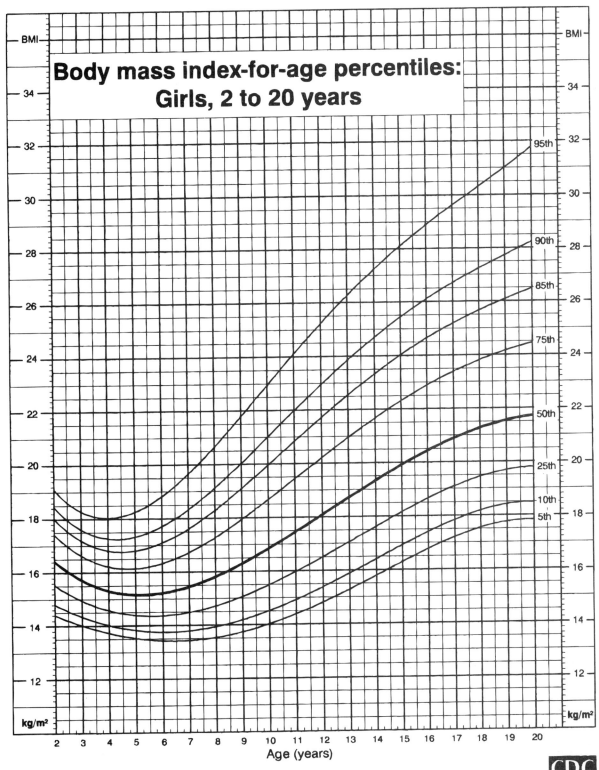

Body mass index-for-age percentiles:
Girls, 2 to 20 years

Published May 30, 2000.
SOURCE: Developed by the National Center for Health Statistics in collaboration with
the National Center for Chronic Disease Prevention and Health Promotion (2000).

CDC
SAFER · HEALTHIER · PEOPLE™

CDC Growth Charts: United States

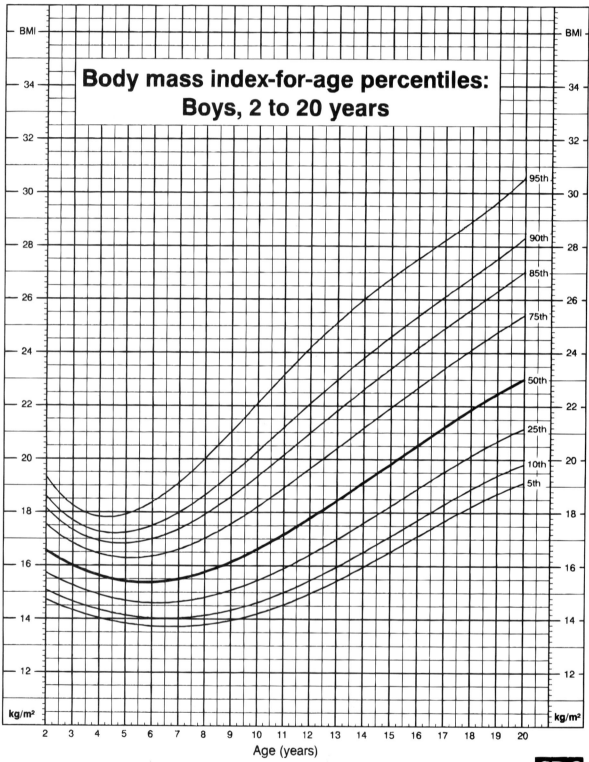

**Body mass index-for-age percentiles:
Boys, 2 to 20 years**

Age (years)

Published May 30, 2000.
SOURCE: Developed by the National Center for Health Statistics in collaboration with
the National Center for Chronic Disease Prevention and Health Promotion (2000).

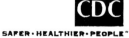

SAFER·HEALTHIER·PEOPLE™

Gross Motor Developmental Milestones for Three Year Old Children

Name _____ Date _____

- [ ] walks smoothly forward
- [ ] walks backwards
- [ ] walks sideways
- [ ] walks up stairs, alternating feet, using a handrail for balance
- [ ] walks on a straight line, balancing with difficulty and watches feet
- [ ] walks short distance on tiptoes
- [ ] runs with better control and can now change speed or direction
- [ ] throws a ball overhead
- [ ] tries to catch a large ball
- [ ] kicks a ball forward
- [ ] jumps with both feet, upward
- [ ] jumps with both feet, forward
- [ ] jumps off low objects
- [ ] hops on one foot
- [ ] stands and balances on one foot momentarily
- [ ] pedals a tricycle
- [ ] climbs up and down a small slide by self

Published by Totline. Copyright protected.   1-57029-519-2 *24-Week Health Plan*

Gross Motor Developmental Milestones for Four Year Old Children

Name _____ Date _____

- ☐ walks backwards
- ☐ walks sideways
- ☐ walks a straight line
- ☐ stands and balances on one foot for five seconds
- ☐ hops on either foot
- ☐ hops forward on one foot about three steps on each foot
- ☐ pedals and steers a tricycle skillfully around obstacles
- ☐ jumps over objects six inches high
- ☐ runs, jumps, hops, and skips around obstacles with ease
- ☐ bounces a ball
- ☐ throws a ball
- ☐ catches a bouncing ball
- ☐ catches a thrown ball
- ☐ gallops
- ☐ turns somersaults
- ☐ climbs ladders
- ☐ tries to skip
- ☐ walk downstairs using a handrail and alternating feet
- ☐ swings on a swing, starting by himself and keeping himself going
- ☐ touches toes without bending knees
- ☐ walks skillfully on a straight line

1-57029-549-2 *24-Week Health Plan*

Gross Motor Developmental Milestones for Five Year Old Children

Name _____ Date _____

- [ ] walks backwards quickly
- [ ] walks sideways
- [ ] walks down stairs, alternating feet without using a handrail
- [ ] runs skillfully
- [ ] runs on tiptoe
- [ ] gallops using either foot in the front
- [ ] skips
- [ ] stands on one foot (either foot) with arms folded across chest to a count of ten seconds
- [ ] hops forward on either foot for a distance of two yards
- [ ] walks on a balance beam
- [ ] throws ball overhead
- [ ] catches bounced balls
- [ ] catches balls thrown lightly
- [ ] rides a tricycle skillfully; may show interest in riding a bicycle with training wheels
- [ ] moves rhythmically to music
- [ ] jumps over low objects
- [ ] jumps over several low objects in a row
- [ ] jumps rope
- [ ] shows interest in performing tricks like standing on head, performing dance steps
- [ ] shows interest in learning complex body coordination skills like swimming, dancing, ice or roller skating, and riding bicycles

Published by Totline. Copyright protected.
1-57029-519-2 *24-Week Health Plan*

Gross Motor Developmental Milestones for Six Year Old Children

Name _____ Date _____

- [ ] jumps rope
- [ ] roller-skates
- [ ] plays hopscotch
- [ ] plays with a Hula-Hoop™
- [ ] runs skillfully
- [ ] runs on tiptoe
- [ ] jumps over several low objects in a row
- [ ] walks forward in a straight line heel-to-toe
- [ ] walks backwards in a straight line heel-to-toe
- [ ] hops on either foot more than 10 times
- [ ] climbs on outdoor jungle gym and play equipment
- [ ] kicks a soccer ball with a greater degree of accuracy
- [ ] rides a bicycle with ease
- [ ] catches a tennis ball using both hands
- [ ] does simple household chores such as sweeping floor or steps
- [ ] shows interest in performing tricks like standing on head, performing dance steps
- [ ] shows interest in learning complex body coordination skills like swimming, dancing, ice or roller skating, and riding bicycles

Name _____ Birthday _____

As you observe the students in your class keep an accurate record of their achievements. Share this checklist with children's parents at appropriate times throughout the health plan activities.

Gross Motor Skill	Date Mastered
walks smoothly forward	
walks backward	
walks up steps, alternating feet	
walks on straight line	
walks short distance on tiptoe	
kicks ball forward	
jumps with both feet, upward	
jumps with both feet forward	
stands still on one foot	
pedals and steers a tricycle	
bounces a ball	
walks downstairs	
hops on one foot	
jumps over low objects	
shows interest in learning dance steps	
turns somersaults	
climbs on jungle gym	
tosses a ball with accuracy	
catches a ball with two hands	
moves rhythmically to music	

Introduction to the First Month of the Health Plan

The first month of *The 24-Week Health Plan* is to introduce the children to the food pyramid recently recreated by the United States Department of Agriculture (UDSA). The children will learn to recognize and sort foods into each of the five food groups (grains, vegetables, fruits, milk, meat and beans). They will be given encouragement and numerous opportunities to try new foods. The children will learn to recognize and realize the importance of well-balanced meals. They will begin to analyze and evaluate the meals that they eat on a daily basis.

In addition children will be introduced and encouraged to participate in daily physical activity. The children will begin to recognize the importance of daily stretching, exercising, and gross motor movement to overall good health. Children will also be working to develop and practice new physical skills. Incorporate the following skills during playtime:

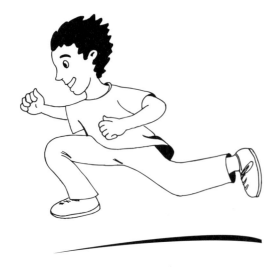

- walking frontward, backward, and sideways on a chalk line
- walking up and down stairs, using alternate feet
- jumping, with both feet
- running during games

Monthly Center

Set up an area to serve as a classroom grocery store. Collect a variety of non-perishable food items (cans of vegetables, soup, boxes of pasta, cereal, macaroni and cheese). The items that are usually purchased in boxes can be empty. Also, gather and display a variety of fruits and vegetables, both real and plastic. Dairy items for the grocery store can include empty and washed out milk cartons, plastic milk jugs, tubs from margarine and/or butter, empty and washed out bags or boxes of cheese. The meat department can be stocked with clean, unused foam meat trays.

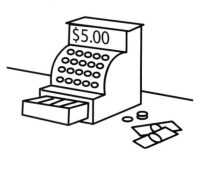

Display a food pyramid prominently in the grocery store. Additionally, a toy cash register, paper, pencils, and pens will also facilitate the children to write grocery lists that include all of the items from the food pyramid.

Suggested activities, lessons, and games are included in *Week One* through *Week Four*. A letter to the parents, *A Tasting Diary*, and *Food Tasting Rules* should be copied and sent home to reinforce the concepts about healthy food choice that are introduced at school.

Dear Parents,

We are starting a 24-week long health program in our classroom. The children will be learning about the importance of nutrition, exercising, and stretching.

This month we will be learning about the food groups as presented in the newest version of the Food Pyramid. The children will learn how each type of food helps us maintain good health. Although many children would rather survive on macaroni and cheese and chicken nuggets and are reluctant to try new foods, they will be encouraged to try new foods from each food group. Research has shown that encouraging children to taste new foods is essential to building a healthy diet. Because children begin to develop their adult food preferences and eating habits around ages four and five, introducing new food during these years will help children increase the variety of foods they will eat during their lifetime.

The following ideas will be introduced in class and can be reinforced at home:

- Follow the "One New Food at a Time" rule. Offer only one new food at a time. This will increase the probability that the new food will be tasted.

- Follow the "Just a Taste" rule. A taste can be as small as a $\frac{1}{2}$ teaspoon. Allow your child to determine the amount to be tasted. All family members should take a taste!

- Follow the "What Goes in May Come Out... and That's Just Fine" rule. Children will be more willing to try a new food if they have the option of spitting it out in a napkin rather than swallowing it.

- Use the "Try, Try Again" rule. Although your child may be reluctant to try new food, continue encouraging and offering nutritious choices. Some research suggests that children may need to be offered the same new food eight to ten times before they will try it.

- Have your child keep a "New Food Journal." List the new foods that are tasted and have your child draw pictures to illustrate them.

In addition, the following gross motor skills will be incorporated into our playtime:

- walking frontward, backward, and sideways on a chalk line

- walking up and down stairs, using alternate feet

Together, we can encourage our children to try and enjoy new food and participate in daily physical activities thus increasing the probability of leading a healthy life!

Sincerely,

Food Is Like a Battery!

This lesson will draw a comparison that food is as important to us as a battery is to a battery-operated toy! Both act as an energy source!

Materials

Battery-operated toy

Batteries

Pretend food or pictures of food

Preparation

Remove batteries from the toy.

Lesson

1. Show the children your battery-operated toy. Tell the children what the toy can do. Turn it on. Exclaim, "Hey! It's not working! I wonder what's wrong with it!"

2. Ask the children if they know what is wrong with your toy. A child will no doubt tell you that maybe it needs new batteries. At this point, retrieve the batteries, put them in and turn the toy on.

3. Talk about how the toy moves around and operates when it has batteries. Ask the children why they think the toy didn't work without batteries.

Tell the children that healthy foods are like batteries for people. Explain that healthy food gives us energy to move around and do our thing. Talk about how we all have a lot of energy in the morning when we first get to school if we have eaten a good and healthy breakfast. Have children think about how they might become a little tired right before lunch, when their "batteries" are running out of energy and they need to eat lunch.

Introduce the Food Pyramid to the children. Tell them that scientists study healthy food and people's bodies for a long time to learn what kind and amount of food people should eat each day. Discuss the different food groups. Put the pretend food or the pictured food where the children can see them. Lead the class in a discussion about the names of the food items and have them work together to decide which food group the foods would be a part of.

Materials

Variety of food from the grocery store center (page 23)

Grocery bags

USDA Food Pyramid Poster (available for download at

http://teamnutrition.usda.gov/Resources/mpk poster2.pdf)

Lesson

1. Review what the children know about the USDA Food Pyramid.

2. Tell the children that they will all have the opportunity to "shop" or "work" at the "grocery store."

3. Choose several children to work at the store acting as cashiers, grocery baggers, produce manager, meat department manager, etc. Choose several children to go to the store and "buy" three items. The items that they purchase must all be from different food groups that are a part of the pyramid.

4. After the children have all had a chance to either work at the store or shop, gather the children together to discuss the purchases. Lead the children in a discussion about the items that were purchased. Have the children discuss which food group the food items are a part of and whether or not they have ever tasted these foods.

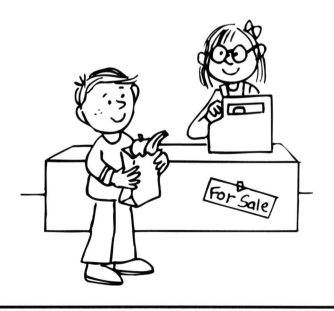

Exercises, Stretches, and Movement Activities

Walk Across the Bridge

Use chalk to draw several sets of straight, double lines with varying widths. Have the children practice walking across the bridge frontward, backward, and shuffling their feet sideways. Have the children walk in this manner on progressively narrower bridges. Encourage the children to walk slowly and quickly.

Challenge the children to walk across the bridge with their arms stretched out at their sides and then change to with their arms down.

Circus Acts!

Use chalk to draw several tightropes on the ground. Encourage the children to pretend to be in a circus and to travel across the tightropes by walking frontward, backward, and shuffling their feet sideways. Encourage the children to walk slowly and quickly. For fun, you can make a longer, wavy tightrope for the children to walk across.

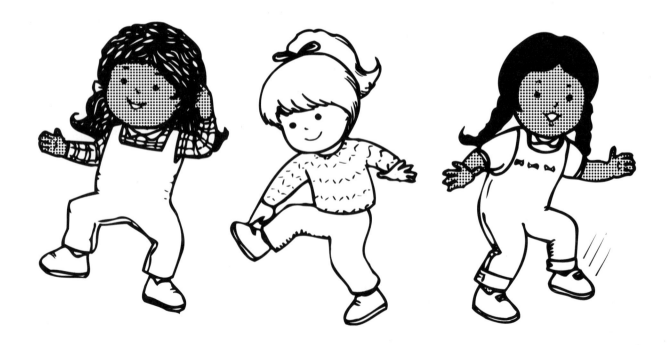

Cut apart the sections below to make a book. Staple the pages together. Draw a picture of each food that you try. Color the face that shows how you feel about the new food.

My Tasting Diary	**I tasted** _____.
I tasted _____.	**I tasted** _____.
I tasted _____.	**I tasted** _____.

Recipe: Food Pyramid Kabobs

Ingredients

Cooked and cooled pasta such as ziti, penne, or shells

Fruit (cut into small chunks) such as apples, pineapple, grapes, bananas

Lightly steamed vegetables (cut into small chunks) such as cucumber, carrots, broccoli, and tomato

Cheese cubes

Cooked chicken, turkey, beef chunks

Wooden skewers

Paper plates

Directions

1. Explain that a "kabob" is made by sticking the wooden skewer through a variety of different foods. It is then often cooked over a fire on an outside barbeque grill. Explain that the food choices that you have supplied have already been cooked, so a grill is not needed.

2. Show the children the food choices. Lead them in a discussion about the different food items. Have the children tell which food group each of the items is part of. Demonstrate how to make a kabob by preparing one yourself. Show the children how to slide the food items onto the skewer.

3. Give each child a paper plate and have the children gather a selection of food. Challenge and encourage the children to select foods from each of the food groups.

4. After the children have made their kabobs, have them tell what food groups are represented on their kabobs.

5. Finally, have the children eat their kabobs. Then have them document the experience in their Tasting Diary (see page 28).

This recipe contains ingredients from the following food groups:

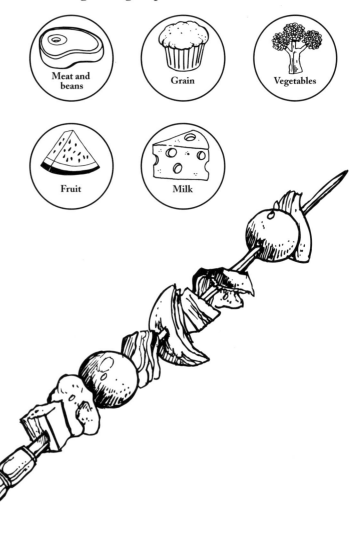

Meat and beans   Grain   Vegetables

Fruit   Milk

Discuss how important running and playing are to the human body. Explain that the more people move their bodies, the stronger and healthier they will be. Tell the children that an added bonus for being active is that the more active a person is the more energy that person will have.

The Bunny Hop

Warm your bunnies up by having them bend their knees and squat down low to the floor. Repeat this several times. Then have your bunnies stretch their legs by standing on their tiptoes and trying to reach the sky without letting their feet leave the ground.

Arrange the children in your circle time area. Have the children pretend to be baby bunnies just learning to hop. Have them practice small hops around in a circle. Next, have the bunnies grow up. Now their hops can be bigger and stronger. Have the grown up bunnies practice

their hops by jumping around the playground. If possible, have them hop out to the playground.

In the playground, designate an area to be the bunnies' home. Designate another area to be the neighbor's garden. Have the bunnies use small hops to move themselves from their home to the neighbor's garden. After the bunnies have rested have them use big, strong hops to go back from the garden to home.

The bunnies should cool off by repeating the warm up stretches. Then lead them in a discussion about which bunny hop was easier and which bunny hop moved them from one place to the other in a quicker manner.

This exercise will help the children develop coordination and gross-motor abilities while strengthening their cardiovascular health.

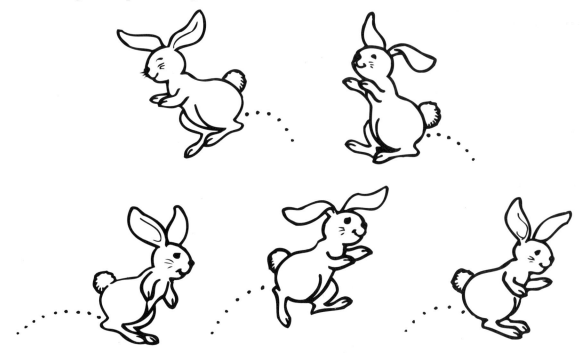

Food Tasting Rules

Make copies of this poster for the children and encourage them to hang them in a prominent place where they can see them while they eat.

1. One new food at a time!

2. Just a taste!

3. What goes in may come out…and that's just fine!

4. Try, try again!

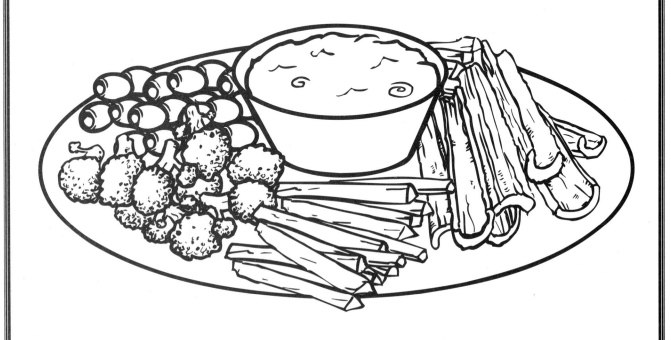

The children will recognize that they are getting daily exercise during their active play both at school and home.

Materials

Chart paper

Construction paper

Crayons

Markers

Lesson

1. Explain that getting enough exercise is important to keep our bodies healthy. Assure the children that they are getting exercise all the time without even thinking of it. Explain that just being active, like running around outside, playing kickball, and climbing trees are all examples of exercise. Explain that playing sports, dancing, doing push-ups, and even walking to and from the car at a store are also forms of exercise.

2. Have the children name activities that they enjoy each day. Write the list on chart paper or on the board. Re-read the list and draw a heart shape next to each activity that counts as exercise.

3. Then give each child a piece of construction paper and crayons or markers. Have the children draw pictures of their favorite exercise. Remind the children that there are many kinds of exercise and that play is the main kind of exercise that most children do. Talk about the differences that they may notice between adult exercises and the types of activities that are more appropriate for children their age.

4. Display these pictures on a bulletin board titled "Play is Exercise!" The pages can also be bound into a book with the same title, then read to the class and stored in the classroom library.

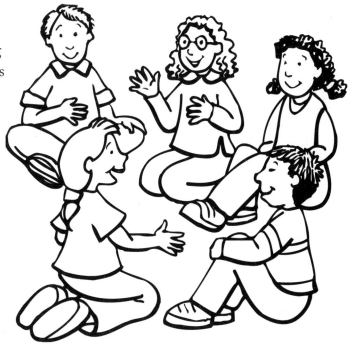

Recipe: Peanut Butter and Banana Wrap

This recipe makes 20 servings.

Ingredients

20 whole wheat tortillas (regular flour tortillas may be used)

Peanut butter

7 bananas

Other Materials

Electric skillet

Paper plates

Napkins

Plastic knives

Directions

1. Heat an electric skillet to a medium temperature.
2. Have the children help you cut bananas into small slices.
3. Give each child a tortilla and a plastic knife. Have each child spread peanut butter on the tortilla.
4. Have the children put banana slices on top of the peanut butter.
5. Lay one peanut butter and banana flour tortilla at a time in the skillet to warm it.
6. When the tortilla is warm and the peanut butter is "melty," help the child roll the tortilla up.

Serve immediately.

This recipe contains ingredients from the following food groups:

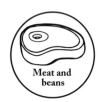
Meat and beans

Fruit

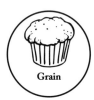
Grain

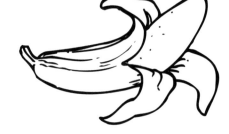

Exercises, Stretches, and Movement Activities

Lead the class in a discussion about how important exercise is when we want to be healthy. Explain that people should spend at least 30 minutes everyday stretching their bodies and exercising or engaging in active play. Have the children name some ways that they enjoy getting physical.

Explain the importance of stretching our muscles to warm them up before engaging in active activities. Tell the children that even animals stretch. They stretch to keep their muscles loose and toned. They stretch to relax after physical exercise or play. Try some of these animal stretches!

The Cat Stretch

Pretend to be an angry cat. Get down on your hands and knees. Arch your back and try to make your back reach up to the ceiling! Then flatten your back. Repeat this five times.

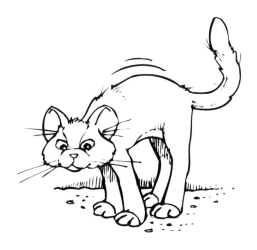

The Turtle Stretch

Stand up straight. Now pretend you are a turtle pulling its head back into its shell by shrugging your shoulders, trying to raise them up to your ears. Stretch your neck tall to make yourself look like a turtle coming out of its shell. Repeat this five times.

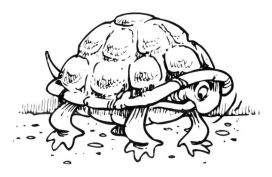

The Snake Stretch

Pretend to be a snake and lay facedown, flat on the floor. Stretch your legs towards one end of the room, trying to touch the wall with your toes. Stretch your arms towards the opposite end of the room, trying to touch the wall with your fingertips. Hold this position and count to five.

The Elephant Stretch

Pretend to be an elephant. Make a trunk by clasping your hands together and straightening your arms. Now reach your trunk down and touch the ground while keeping your knees straight. Next raise your trunk high in the air. Repeat this five times.

Let's Go Shopping!

Materials

Grocery Store Center (page 24)

Card stock

Index cards

Markers

Preparation

Make grocery lists for your students (one list for every two to three students) by cutting out food pictures or using images from this book and gluing three or four items to index cards. Laminate for durability.

Lesson

1. Divide the class into pairs or small groups. Explain that you will be sending them to the grocery store to pick up several items.

2. Give each pair or group a grocery lists. Have the children take turns going to store and picking up the items.

3. When all of the children have selected their items, have the groups take turns naming the food items and sharing whether or not they have tried the food item.

4. After all of the groups have had a turn to talk about their food, have the children work together to sort the food items into the different food groups (Meat and Bean, Dairy, Fruit, Vegetable, and Grains).

Finally, have the children answer the following questions:

- How many items are in each of the Pyramid food groups?
- Which food group had the most items in it?
- Which food group had the least amount of items in it?

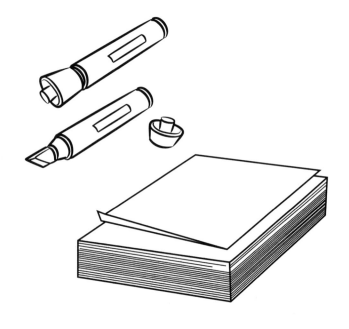

This recipe makes 20 small servings.

Ingredients

1 dozen eggs

$\frac{1}{2}$ teaspoon salt

$\frac{1}{8}$ teaspoon pepper

$\frac{3}{4}$ cup milk

3 tablespoons butter

This recipe contains ingredients from the following food groups:

Meat and beans

Fats, oils, and sweets

Milk

Directions

1. Mix the eggs, salt, pepper, and milk in the mixing bowl. Make sure the egg mixture is beaten well and that all ingredients are mixed.

2. In a large skillet, melt 3 tablespoons butter or margarine over medium heat.

3. Pour in the egg mixture and stir occasionally until the eggs are semi-hardened and fully cooked.

4. Serve immediately.

NOTE: By adding 2/3 cup of shredded mild Cheddar cheese or American cheese to the egg mixture, you can make cheesy eggs that taste even better. Or cut up ham or turkey slices and add it to the egg mixture to give the snack even more of a protein punch.

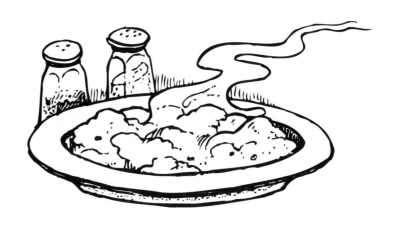

Nature's Movement and Exercises

Jump On Your Shadow!

One of the most interesting things about shadows is that a person is unable to jump directly on his or her own shadow. Children will try for long period of time when challenged to successfully complete this task. Have the children stand in a straight line out in the open sunlight. Make sure there is space between each child so they can have fun trying to step on themselves. Instruct them to jump to the left, to the right, frontward, and backward. Have them run up, trying to "sneak" up to their shadows. Challenge the children to find anyway possible to step on their own shadows.

Shadow Tag

Choose three or four children to be "it." Their job is to tag other children's shadows. Once a child's shadow has been tagged, that child has to freeze. When all of the remaining children's shadows have been tagged, choose new children to be "it."

Shadow Climb

Find the shadow of a tree or of the jungle gym. Challenge the children to show you how to climb the tree's shadow. Be sure that the children use their arms and legs as they climb.

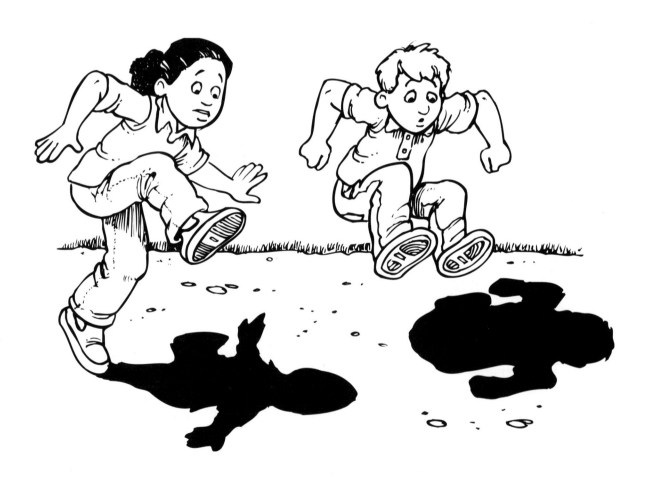

Introduction to the Second Month of the Health Plan

The goal of this second month of the 24-Week Health Plan is to familiarize the children with foods that are included in the grain group. The children will be having opportunities to try foods and learn how to estimate correct portion sizes for the grain group. The children will learn that grains are the foods that give us energy and that they are an important part of well-balanced meals. They will begin to analyze and self evaluate the grain products that they eat on a daily basis.

The children will be encouraged to continue daily physical activity. They will recognize the importance of daily stretching, exercising, and gross motor movement for overall good health. Please incorporate the following skills into playtime:

- Running during games
- Walking or running on tip-toes
- Dancing rhythmically to music
- Jumping up, with both feet
- Balancing on one foot

Monthly Center

Set up an area in the classroom to serve as a classroom bakery. Collect a variety of boxes of pasta, cereal, and macaroni and cheese. Include modeling dough, a rolling pin, and cookie cutters in the center so that the children can make bread, rolls, cookies, and cake.

Suggested activities, lessons, and games are included in *Weeks Five* through *Eight*. A letter to the parents, *A Tasting Diary, Look at My Serving Size, Eat Your Grains*, and *Family Project: My Family Pasta Creation* should be copied and sent home to reinforce concepts about eating healthy grains that are introduced at school.

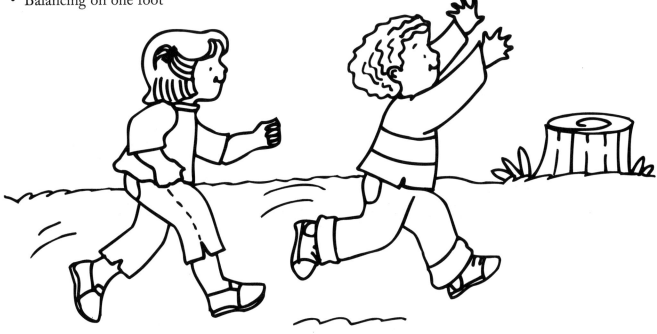

Parent Letter, Weeks 5–8

Dear Parents:

The children were kept very busy during month one, learning about the food pyramid, new stretches, and playing games that help them work up a sweat. This month, the following gross motor skills will be incorporated into our playtime:

- Running during games
- Walking or running on tiptoes
- Dancing rhythmically to music
- Jumping up, with both feet
- Balancing on one foot

Please encourage your child to practice these gross motor skills at home.

Our food focus will be even more specific information about the grain group. The new USDA food pyramid recommends eating at least six ounces of grains each day. They also suggest making at least three ounces of your grains whole grains.

An easy solution to this issue is cereal! One cup of nutritious cereal will supply almost half the daily nutritional requirements for important vitamins and minerals. Since most children enjoy adding milk, another food group is represented in the meal and the nutritional content is even higher. Most cereals are loaded with sugar; however a recent study by the *Journal of the American Dietetic Association* found that teenage girls who regularly ate cereal with breakfast weighed less than girls who skipped breakfast. Recent studies have shown children who eat breakfast every day perform better, tend to make healthier food choices throughout the day, and are more likely to participate in physical activities.

It is often necessary to eat breakfast "on the run." Some suggestions are:

- Breakfast tacos or burritos
- Bananas and peanut butter on a hotdog bun
- Cream cheese and fruit on a bagel or pita.

We will also continue introducing stretches, exercises, and movement games this month. Have your child demonstrate some of his or her new skills at home!

Have a healthy month!

Sincerely,

Materials

Several medium-sized tubs with covers

A variety of grain products, such as white flour, whole wheat flour, oatmeal, and a variety of dried pastas

Measuring cups

Spoons

Funnels

Sifters

Small containers such as plastic cups or bowls

Lesson:

1. Read a book about foods from the grain food group (see the book list).

2. Lead the children in a discussion about the story. Have the children name examples of the different foods mentioned in the book that are part of the grain group.

3. Show the children the tub containing pasta, white rice, or brown rice. Open the top and have the children look at what is inside. Have the children discuss whether or not they have ever eaten the food that is in the tub.

4. Open another tub containing cornmeal, white flour, whole wheat flour, or oatmeal. Ask the children if they recognize what is in the tub. Have the children name the ingredient and tell what it can be used to cook.

5. Continue opening each tub and discussing its contents.

6. Then display the measuring cups, spoons, funnels, and sifter. Discuss their experiences with these items.

7. Take the children outside and allow them to experiment with the variety of grain products using the measuring cups and other kitchen items.

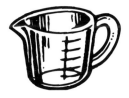

Recipe: Popcorn Delight

This recipe makes 24 cups.

Ingredients

8 ounces unpopped popcorn

4 tablespoon butter or margarine, melted

4 tablespoons honey

$\frac{1}{2}$ teaspoon cinnamon

2 cups raisins or peanuts (or 1 cup of each)

Other materials

Air popcorn popper or pot, heat source, and oil

Disposable cups to serve popcorn

2-13 x 9 inch baking pans

Directions

1. Preheat oven to 275°F.
2. Pop the popcorn according to the directions on the package.
3. Divide the popped popcorn and put some in each of two 13 x 9-inch baking pans.
4. Combine the melted butter, honey, and cinnamon. Pour over the popcorn and stir until evenly coated.
5. Bake for 10 minutes. Spread the popcorn on foil to cool.
6. Stir in the raisins and/or peanuts.

This recipe contains ingredients from the following food groups:

Grain

Meat and beans

Fats, oils, and sweets

Fruit

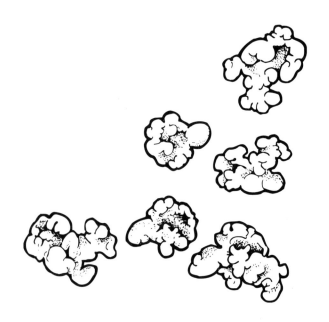

Enjoy working out and stretching with Hansel and Gretel.

Hansel and Gretel

Use bread crumbs to make a long trail on the playground. Take the children outside and show them the bread trail. Ask them if it reminds them of a story. Talk about which food group the bread crumbs belong to. Choose two children to pretend to be Hansel and Gretel. Have Hansel and Gretel agree on a way to move along the trail. Have the rest of the children follow them as they move along the trail. Some examples of locomotion are:

- run
- walk
- crawl
- jump
- skip

Hansel and Gretel Stretch Out Their Arms

Hansel and Gretel took a long walk. They were careful to leave a trail of bread crumbs. Their arms were sore because of bending and straightening their arms as they tore and placed the bread crumbs on the ground. When they rested they stretched their arms.

You can stretch your arms like Hansel and Gretel:

- Stretch your right arm straight out in front of you. With your left hand, hold the top of your right arm (do not hold your elbow) and pull it gently across your body. Hold for five seconds. Repeat with the other arm.

- Raise your right hand up in the air with your upper arm near your ear. Bend your elbow and let your right fore arm hang near your back. Use your left arm to grasp your upper arm and gently pull it towards the middle of your body. Hold it for five seconds. Repeat with the other arm.

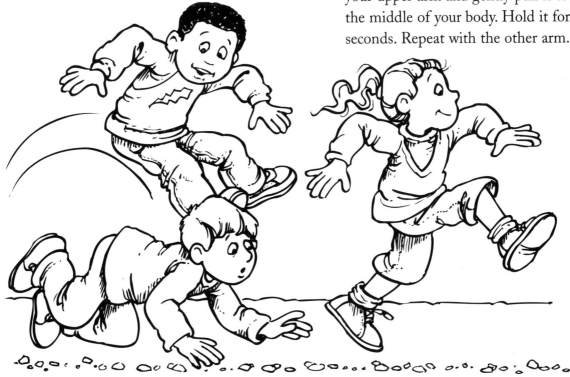

Look at My Serving Size!

Directions:

You can eat your daily requirement of grains in many ways! Draw and color these favorite grains. See if you are eating the right amount.

Serving Size of Grain	Equals This Easy-to-Use Comparison
slice bread	**1 grain serving, same as a slice of bread**
$\frac{1}{2}$ cup rice	**1 serving, same size as a tennis ball**
$\frac{1}{2}$ cup oatmeal	**1 serving, same size as a tennis ball**
1 ounce dry cereal	**1 serving, same as one adult handful**
1 bagel	**1 serving, same size as a hockey puck**
1 muffin or dinner roll	**1 serving, same size as a fist**

Materials

Little Red Hen by Paul Galdone
(Clarion Books, 1985)

Props to act out the story, such as gardening tools, seeds, bowls, and spoons

Lesson and Activity

1. Read *Little Red Hen* to the children. Have the children retell their favorite parts.

2. Point out all of the steps that have to occur in order to bake bread. Have the children name the things that the Little Red Hen did during the story. Make a list of their suggestions. Then, have the children order the steps in the correct order.

3. Tell the children that they are going to act out the story. Choose one child for each of the following parts: Little Red Hen, Duck, Dog, and Cat.

4. Read the story again and have the children say their dialogue and act out their parts.

5. Finally, store the book in the Dramatic Play Area. Encourage the children to act out the story during their free time.

An easy recipe for bread can be found on page 46 and is a good follow-up to this lesson!

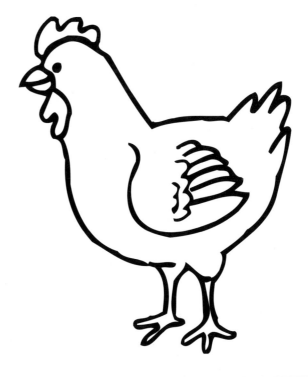

Recipe: Easy Oatmeal Bread

Ingredients

1 packet yeast

2 tablespoons molasses or honey

1 cup rolled oats

1 tablespoon butter plus $\frac{1}{2}$ t. for buttering pan

1 teaspoon salt

1 cup unbleached flour plus $\frac{1}{2}$ cup for kneading

1 cup whole wheat flour

Directions

1. In a mixing bowl, combine yeast, molasses, and 1 cup warm water (wrist temperature). Let sit until yeast is bubbly (about 5 minutes). Stir in oats and butter and let sit for 5 minutes.

2. Add salt and flours, stirring in $\frac{1}{2}$ cup at a time. Knead dough into a soft blob, return it to the bowl, and cover with a damp cloth. Let rise until double in bulk (about 30 minutes).

3. Punch dough down and knead until smooth, adding reserved flour as needed.

4. Shape into a loaf, place in a buttered loaf pan, cover again, and let rise. When loaf has doubled in bulk again, place in the oven and bake at 350°F until done (about 45 minutes). Cool on a rack for 15 minutes before slicing.

This recipe contains ingredients from the following food groups:

Grain Group, including whole grains

Oils

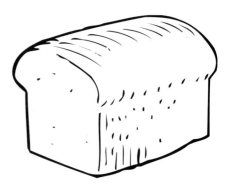

Exercises, Stretches, and Movement Activities

Flamingo Stand

Have the children pretend to be resting flamingos. Flamingos rest by balancing on one foot. Children will stand on one foot, while bending the resting leg at the knee. Challenge the children to rest like flamingos for five seconds, then ten seconds. Have the children switch legs and try balancing on the other foot.

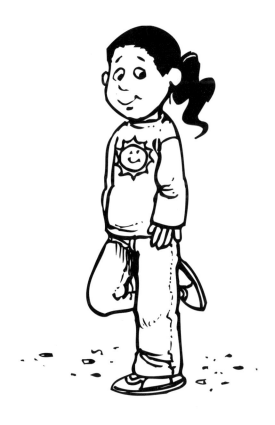

Document balancing times on a chart. With practice, the balancing times will increase!

Note: This activity will help the children increase their ability to balance on one foot. Developing balance is essential because it is used for so many large muscle (gross motor) activities.

The Flamingo Stretch

Demonstrate the flamingo stretch by standing on one foot, while bending your left leg at the knee. Hold on to a chair for balance. Reach back with your left hand and hold your foot. Gently pull your foot towards the back of your leg. Hold this position for ten seconds. Repeat this with your right leg. Stretch each leg three times.

Explain that this position stretches out the quadriceps muscle.

Ocean Motion

Take the children outside. Invite the children to pretend that they are floating in the ocean on a calm day. Tell them that there are no big waves, just small ones. Next tell them to pretend the ocean is wild! Have them to pretend that they are the huge waves that are crashing on the beach!

Next, divide the children into two groups. Put the two groups on either side of the playground. One half of the children will pretend that they are playing on the beach. Have the other half will pretend to be the waves. When you shout, "GO!" the children playing should run towards the "waves." When you shout, "Waves splash!" the playing children should turn around and run the other way while the "waves" try to tag them. The children who are tagged will become "waves."

Eat Your Grains!

Keep track of the grains that you eat this week. Color one slice of bread for each serving you eat each day. Color your whole grains with a brown crayon.

Monday
Grains...6 a day

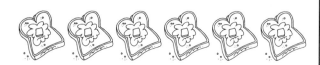

Tuesday
Grains...6 a day

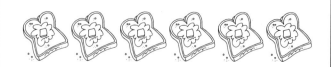

Wednesday
Grains...6 a day

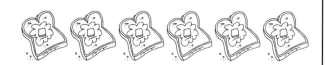

Thursday
Grains...6 a day

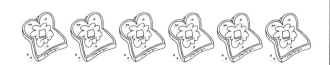

Friday
Grains...6 a day

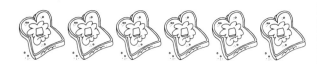

Saturday
Grains...6 a day

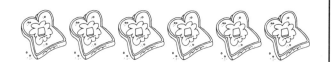

Sunday
Grains...6 a day

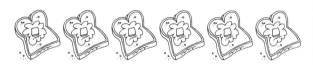

Remember that grains include:

breakfast cereal, bread, rice, pasta, oatmeal, cornmeal, bagel, English muffin

Breads From Around the World

Materials

Toaster

Spreads such as butter, jelly or jam,
    cream cheese

Bread such as white, bagels, pitas, tortillas,
    cinnamon bread

Paper plates

Napkins

Plastic knives

Lesson

1. Ask the children what kinds of bread they
   like to eat. After several children have
   shared their favorite kinds of bread, have
   the children respond to the following:

   • Touch your nose if you have ever
     eaten a bagel.

   • Wiggle your fingers if you have ever
     eaten a tortilla.

   • Nod your head if you have ever eaten
     corn bread.

   • Clap your hands one time if you have
     ever eaten Italian bread.

   • Snap your fingers if you have ever eaten
     cinnamon bread.

   • Give thumbs up if you have ever eaten
     pita bread or a pita pocket.

2. Read a recommended book or select other
   books that show and tell about breads from
   around the world. Lead the class in a
   discussion about the breads.

3. Display the variety of bread and spread
   choices. Have each child prepare a snack.
   Then, cut each child's snack in quarters.
   Encourage all of the children to eat one
   quarter of their snacks and trade the
   remaining with friends. This will give the
   children the opportunity to try many new
   kinds of bread.

4. Finally, have the children share their
   thoughts regarding the different kinds of
   bread they sampled. Have the children
   document the new food they tried in a
   Tasting Diary (found on page 29).

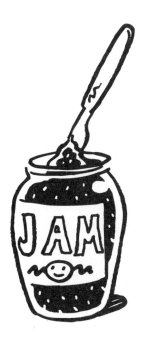

Recipe: Sesame Noodles

This recipe makes 16 one-ounce servings.

Ingredients

1 pound angel hair pasta (or the thinnest pasta available)

$\frac{1}{2}$ cup soy sauce

$\frac{1}{4}$ cup sesame oil

$\frac{1}{3}$ cup sugar

3 scallions, thinly sliced

$\frac{1}{4}$ cup sesame seeds (or more)

Other Materials

Heat source

Large pot

Pasta strainer

Knife

Cutting board

Paper bowls

Forks (or chopsticks)

Directions

1. Thinly slice the scallions and set aside.

2. Mix the soy sauce, sesame oil, and the sugar until it is well blended and the sugar has dissolved.

3. Cook the spaghetti according to the package directions and drain.

4. Pour the sesame sauce over the hot pasta. Toss with scallions and sprinkle with the sesame seeds.

Serve hot and enjoy!

This recipe contains ingredients from the following food groups:

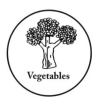
Vegetables

Grain

Fats, oils, and sweets

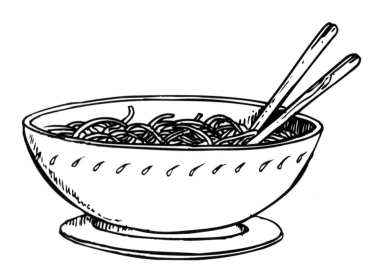

The Spaghetti Dance

Put on some fast music and have the children pretend that they are as wiggly and flexible as a cooked piece of spaghetti! Challenge the children to continue moving until the song is over. After the dance workout, have the children stretch and demonstrate their flexibility. Then put the music on again and have them move. Finish with a cool down stretch.

Have the children pretend to dance like other types of fun pasta. They can spring up and down like corkscrew pasta, lie on the floor and wiggle like lasagna noodles, and stand straight and stretch like linguini.

Popcorn

Teach the children the following chant. Have the children repeat the chant and begin to "pop" like hot popcorn. Encourage as much popping as they can stand. Try to build up to five minutes of popping without a rest.

Popcorn Is My Name

Popcorn, popcorn is my name.

I am one good tasty grain!

Cook me in a microwave or pot,

Once I'm hot, I'll pop, pop, pop!

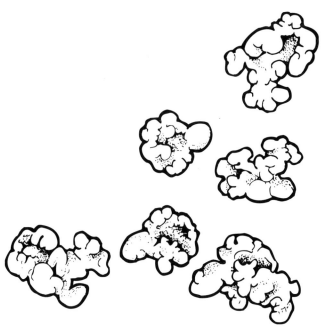

How Much Do I Need?

Materials

Tubs containing grains

Measuring cups

Small, medium, and large bowls

Paper plates

Several tennis balls

One copy of *Look at My Serving Size* (see page 44)

Lesson

1. Lead the class in a discussion about the grain group. Have children name some foods that are from the grain group. Ask the children to explain why it is important for us to include grains in our daily diet. (Grains supply us with the energy necessary for work and play!)

2. Review the proper serving size of grains. Review the *Look at My Serving Size*, page 43.

3. Choose volunteers to fill each of the small, medium, and large bowls with one $\frac{1}{2}$ cup servings of pasta. Lead the class in a discussion about how the serving sizes look different depending on the bowl. Ask the children which bowl they would like to eat pasta from and have them explain why.

4. Show the children a tennis ball. Suggest that they imagine the size of a tennis ball when they are eating a serving of pasta. Explain that if they eat a portion this size, they will be getting a healthy part of their grain serving.

5. Repeat the above activity with rice and oatmeal. Then give the children an opportunity to practice measuring out $\frac{1}{2}$ cup serving sizes (tennis ball servings) of pasta, rice, and oatmeal. Have the children work on measuring the correct portion size and putting the food on a variety of plates.

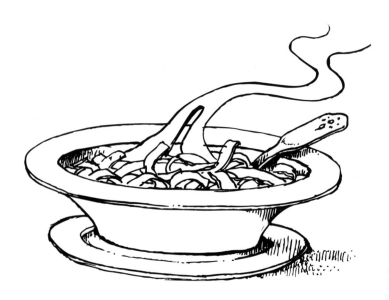

Pasta, Pasta, Pasta!

Materials

Several cooked pasta dishes for the children to sample.

Lesson

Tell the children that they are going to learn about a food from the grain group that is usually very popular with children. Have the children try to guess what kind of grain food you are talking about.

After someone guesses that they are going to learn about pasta, have the children describe their favorite pasta dishes.

Then ask the children if they know what pasta is made out of. Have the children brainstorm a list of possible ingredients. Write the children's suggestions on the board or on chart paper.

Then read one of the recommended books or select another book that shows and tells about the different kinds of pasta and how it is made.

After reading the book, have the children review their list of possible ingredients for making pasta. Have volunteers circle the ingredients that are necessary to make pasta and also to cross off the ingredients that are not a part of a pasta recipe.

Allow the children the opportunity to try the pastas that you have prepared: Have the children share their thoughts regarding the foods they sampled. Have the children document the new food they tried in a Tasting Diary (page 29).

Have the children assist you in making the pasta that they are to sample. Sometimes when children are involved in the preparation, they are more likely to try new food dishes!

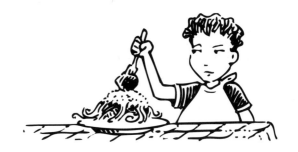

Recipe: Peanut Butter Pasta

This recipe makes 16 one-ounce servings.

Ingredients

8 oz. box linguine (1 package)

2 tablespoons peanut butter

1 teaspoon salt

5 tablespoons soy sauce

2 tablespoons sesame oil

2 teaspoons sugar

1 teaspoon white wine vinegar

2 garlic cloves, minced

2 teaspoons onion, grated or minced

Other Materials

Heat source

Large pot

Pasta strainer

Knife

Cutting Board

Paper bowls

Forks

Directions

Cook linguine according to package instructions in boiling water and then drain. In large bowl, mix all the remaining ingredients together. Add linguine to sauce and toss to coat well.

Serve warm.

This recipe contains ingredients from the following food groups:

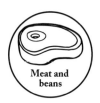

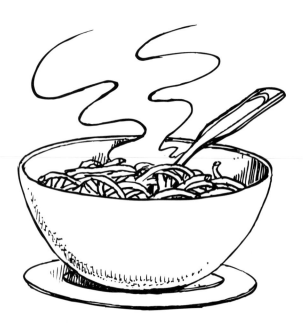

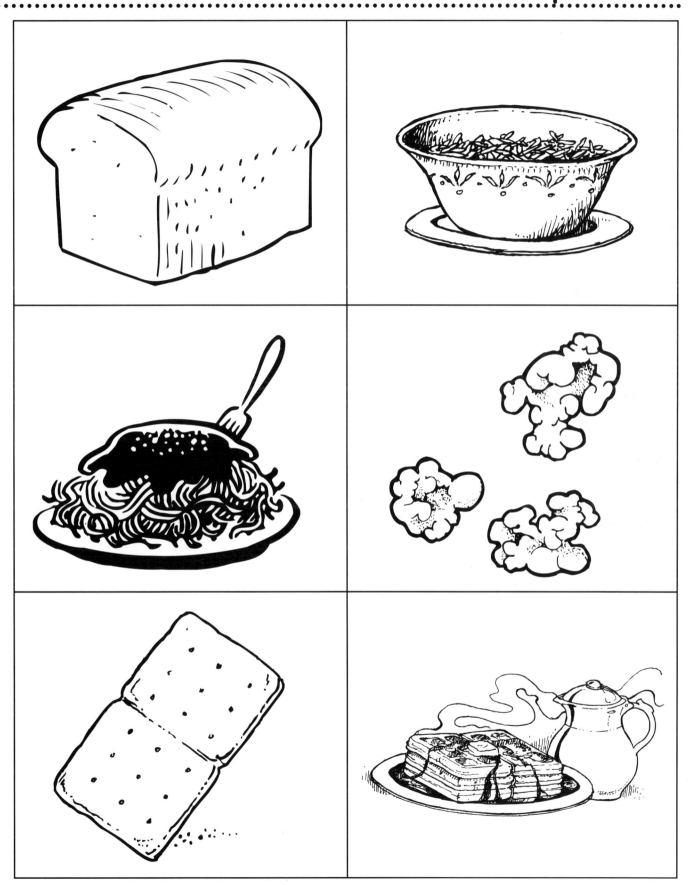

Family Project: My Family Pasta Creation

Family Name _____

Work together with your family to create an interesting pasta dish. Be sure to help with the cooking! Don't forget to add ingredients from as many food groups as you can.

Check off the boxes to show what food groups you included in your pasta dish:

☐ Grain Group

☐ Vegetable Group

☐ Fruit Group

☐ Meat and Bean Group

☐ Dairy Group

☐ Oil

Practice telling about the pasta creation with your family as the audience. Be ready to tell your friends.

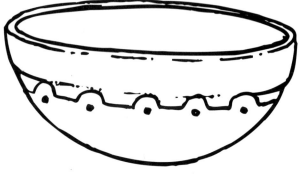

The name of my pasta dish is

_____ .

I tasted my pasta dish and it was

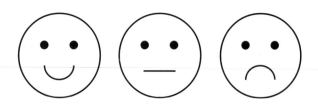

Introduction to the Third Month of the Health Plan

The third month of the *24-Week Health Plan* is about the vegetable group of the Food Pyramid. The children will have the opportunity to try foods and learn how to estimate correct portion sizes for the vegetable group. The children will learn that vegetables supply us with important vitamins and nutrients that help us stay healthy. They will begin to analyze and self evaluate the vegetable products that they eat on a daily basis.

The children will continue to be introduced and encouraged to participate in daily physical activity. Please incorporate the following gross motor skills into playtime:

- Hopping, on either foot
- Galloping, using either foot in the front
- Kicking a ball, using either foot

Monthly Center

Set up an area in the classroom to serve as a classroom vegetable stand. Collect a variety of fresh or plastic vegetables, cans of vegetables, and empty and cleaned packaging from frozen vegetables. In addition, request unused foam trays or baskets from the produce department at the local store. Cut out pictures of vegetables and glue these pictures onto the foam trays. Include a balance scale, a cash register, and bags so the children can pretend to buy and sell the vegetables.

Suggested activities, lessons, and games will be included in *Weeks Nine* through *Twelve*. A letter to the parents, *A Tasting Diary*, and an *Am I Eating My Vegetables*? should be copied and sent home to reinforce the concepts about healthy eating as well as including vegetables in our diets each day.

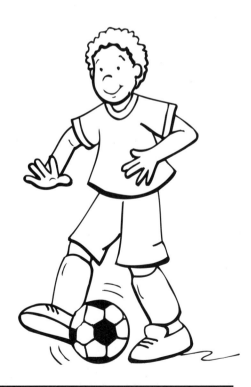

Dear Parents:

The children are enjoying learning about the food pyramid, trying new foods, and incorporating exercise into our daily schedule. Hopefully, the children are following through with what they are learning in school while at home. Ask your child to tell you about the new things he or she has learned about eating and exercising to stay healthy. This third month we will be incorporating the following gross motor activities in our playtime. You can do these at home too.

- Hopping, on either foot

- Galloping, using either foot in the front

- Kicking a ball, using either foot

This month our food focus will be more specific. The children will be learning about the different kinds of food found in the vegetable group. The newest USDA food pyramid recommends eating at least $2\frac{1}{2}$ cups of vegetables each day. They also recommend offering children a variety of different colored vegetables.

Because it is a challenge to get many children to eat vegetables, here are some helpful hints:

- Most children prefer to eat vegetables raw. Carrots, celery, green pepper, cucumber, broccoli, cauliflower, fresh peas, or pea pods can be a crunchy, tasty snack or dinner item.

- Pair raw vegetables with a dip such as ranch dressing, cheese sauce, or mild salsa (which has additional vegetables).

- When cooking vegetables, don't overcook them. Lightly steam or boil them until they are tender but not mushy.

Acknowledge that vegetables may not be a favorite food choice. However, explain that it is important to learn to "enjoy" a variety of foods to maintain health. After all, it is easier to encourage healthy eating habits when children are young than to correct unhealthy eating habits that have been in place for years! Have a healthy month!

Sincerely,

Lessons and Activities for Week Nine: Grow Your Vegetables

Materials

Foam cups

Fork

Soil

Vegetable seeds (available at garden stores)

Preparation

Use the fork to poke several sets of hole in the bottom of each foam cup to allow the extra water to drain.

Directions:

1. Read *From Seed to Plant* by Gail Gibbons or *Growing Vegetable Soup* by Lois Ehlert. Lead the class in a discussion about what they learned.

2. Display the variety of vegetable seeds. Give the children an opportunity to examine the seeds. Tell the children what each seed will produce.

3. Tell the children that they will be able to each plant a seed. Have the children choose the seeds they want to plant. Assist the children, as they write their names on their cups, fill the cup with soil, poke a hole in the soil, insert the seed, and cover the seed with soil.

4. Explain that it is important to supply the seed with water, but that too much water is not good. Point out the holes that you put in the bottom of each cup. Explain that the holes are there so that the extra water can drain out. Demonstrate how to water the seed.

5. Have the children take care of their seeds and discuss the daily growth.

6. When the seeds have grown into a plant, have the children take their plants home and continue to take care of them. Ask the children to keep the class up-to-date about the plant's growth and progress.

Optional: Replant these plants in a garden at school. The children will enjoy harvesting and eating the vegetables that they have grown!

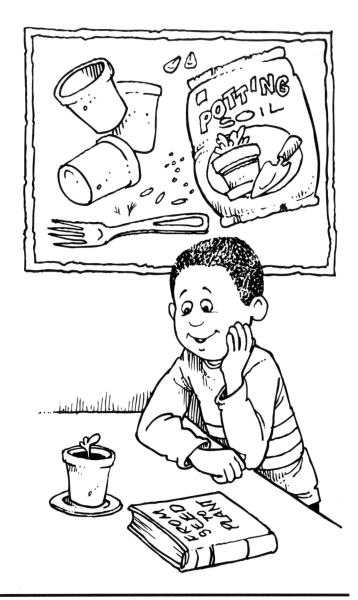

Recipe: Vegetable Dip

This recipe makes about two cups of dip.

Ingredients

1 cup sour cream

1 cup mayonnaise (lite or fat-free)

1 tablespoon lemon juice

1 tablespoon dried chives

$\frac{1}{2}$ teaspoon dill weed

1 teaspoon garlic salt

$\frac{1}{2}$ teaspoon paprika

Vegetables for dipping

Baby carrots

Cucumber slices

Celery sticks

Broccoli spears

Red or yellow peppers, thinly sliced

Directions

Combine all of the ingredients in a small bowl and blend well. Chill the dip in the refrigerator for at least one hour before serving.

This recipe contains ingredients from the following food groups:

Milk

Vegetables

Fats, oils, and sweets

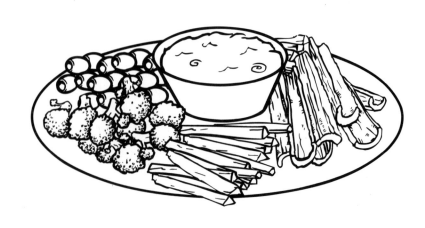

Kick and Chase!

Bring several balls out to the playground. Divide the children into pairs or small groups of three. Have one child kick the ball. The other children will wait until the ball stops rolling and run after (or chase) the ball. When the runners have come to the ball they must freeze and wait until everyone in the group has arrived. Have the children switch positions and continue playing as time allows.

Challenge the children to run not simply in the direction of the ball but in a similar path. If the ball was kicked and it zigzags around on the playground, have the children do the same thing.

Good for You Galloping

Take the children outside and demonstrate how to gallop. Have the children who have mastered this gross motor skill gallop around the playground. Work individually with the children who are still learning. Encourage the children to choose horse names and have informal horse races to encourage galloping.

This activity can be done with skipping or hopping as well.

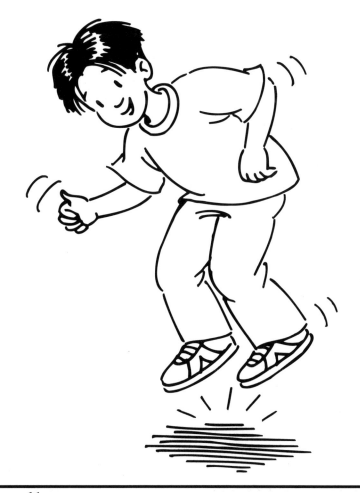

Vegetable Patterns

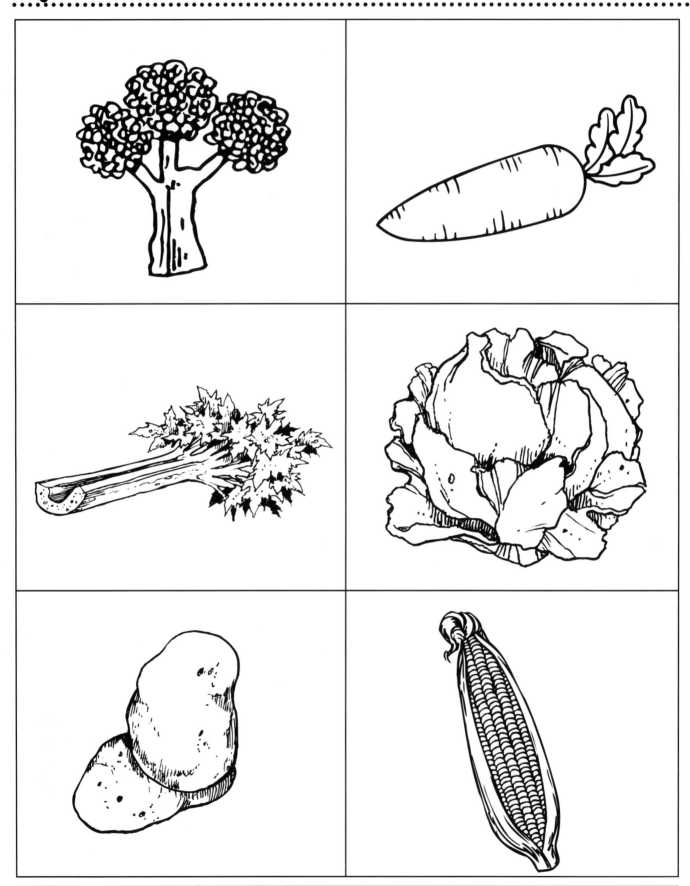

Materials:

Paper plates

Pictures of food

Glue

Crayons

Lesson

Lead the class in a discussion about the new foods that they have tried, both at home and at school.

Discuss how important it is to have all of the food groups represented at each meal. Explain that if they do this, it will be easier to meet the daily recommended requirements.

Show the children the paper plates and the pictures of the food. Challenge the children to prepare a healthy meal by cutting out and coloring the food that they would choose if they were preparing a meal for their families.

Finally, give all of the children an opportunity to show and tell about the meal they have prepared. Have the children tell what food groups are represented in each meal.

Display these meals on a bulletin board titled "Look What We Are Serving!"

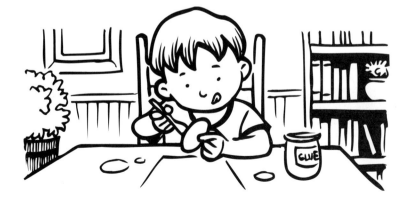

Lessons and Activities for Week Ten: Colorful Veggies

Materials

Chart paper

Variety of vegetables—real, plastic, pictures from magazine or copied and colored pictures (page 61), canned, and empty containers of frozen vegetables

Directions

1. Lead the class in a discussion about their favorite kinds of vegetables. List the children's favorite vegetables on the board or on chart paper.

2. Explain that different colors of vegetables keep us healthy in different ways. Suggest that the children sort the vegetables according to color.

3. Designate areas for each color of vegetable. Have one child at a time choose a vegetable and put it into the appropriate area.

4. After all the children have sorted the vegetables by color, share the following information with the children:

   • The purple and blue vegetables help keep your memory working.

   • The green vegetables help keep your vision, bones, and teeth healthy.

   • The white vegetables keep your heart healthy.

   • The yellow vegetables keep your heart, eyes, and immune system healthy.

   • The red vegetables help to keep your memory and urinary tract healthy.

5. Have the children count the vegetables in each color group. Discuss which color group has the most and least vegetables.

6. Finally, point out how important it is to eat vegetables from each color group, since each of the colors help to keep a different area of our body healthy.

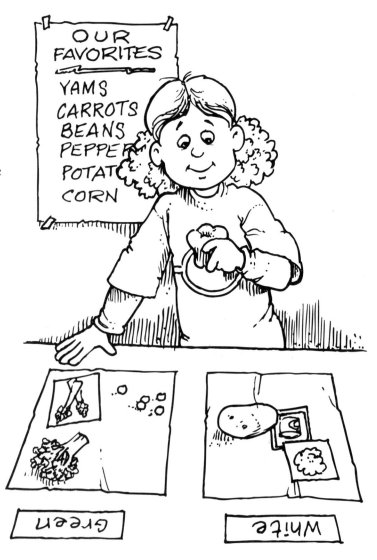

This recipe makes 20 servings.

Ingredients

2 quarts chicken broth

2 chopped yellow onions

16 ounces cream cheese (2 blocks)

8 cups sliced zucchini

Salt and pepper to taste

This recipe contains ingredients from the following food groups:

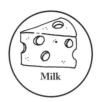 Milk

 Meat and beans

 Vegetables

Directions

1. Put one cup of chicken broth and the chopped vegetables into a pot and cover. Cook until vegetables are tender.

2. Add the cream cheese and stir until the cheese is melted.

3. Put the mixture in a blender and puree.

4. Return the mixture to the pot. Add the rest of the chicken broth and stir.

5. Add salt and pepper to taste and then serve.

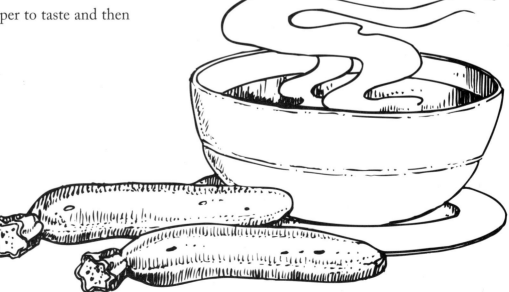

Exercises, Stretches, and Movement Activities

Fitness Soup

In the story, *Stone Soup*, the characters are fooled into sharing their food to create delicious soup that feeds all of the hungry people in the town. "Fitness Soup" can be made when each child takes a turn teaching the class an exercise, stretch, or movement of his or her choice. After each child has had a chance to lead the class in his or her fitness activity, the class will have enjoyed "Fitness Soup!"

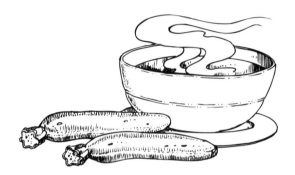

Weed your Garden!

Have the children pretend that they have planted a vegetable garden. Have them pretend to take care of their gardens by doing the following:

Do a set of five squats to pull the weeds from their garden by standing with their feet shoulder length apart and their hands on their hips. They will bend their knees at a 90 degree angle, making sure that their knees do not extend over the end of their feet (keep the knees at a 90 degree angle to avoid injury). Repeat three times.

Do a set of five jumping jacks, encouraging the plants in the garden to grow big and tall. Begin with arms at their sides. As children swing their arms above their heads to clap, they must jump up and spread their feet about shoulder width apart.

After weeding, gardeners need to relax. Have the children sit cross-legged on the floor. Have them place their hands in their laps and take five deep breaths, in and out.

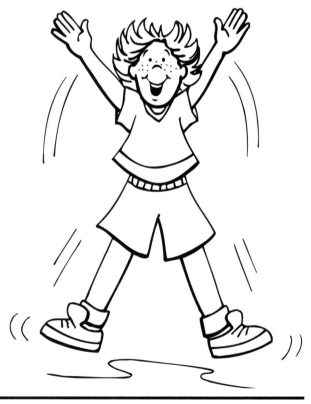

Keep track of the vegetables that you eat this week! Remember, vegetables supply us with many vitamins and nutrients that keep our bodies healthy. Color your vegetables.

Monday
Vegetables...2 $\frac{1}{2}$ cups a day

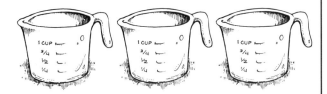

Tuesday
Vegetables...2 $\frac{1}{2}$ cups a day

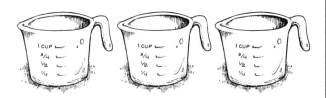

Wednesday
Vegetables...2 $\frac{1}{2}$ cups a day

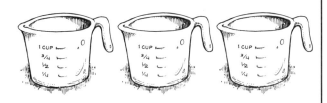

Thursday
Vegetables...2 $\frac{1}{2}$ cups a day

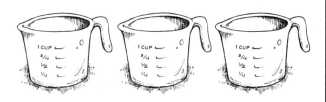

Friday
Vegetables...2 $\frac{1}{2}$ cups a day

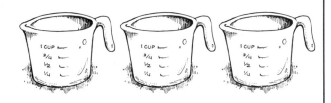

Saturday
Vegetables...2 $\frac{1}{2}$ cups a day

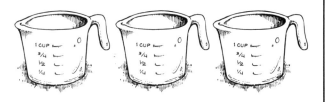

Sunday
Vegetables...2 $\frac{1}{2}$ cups a day

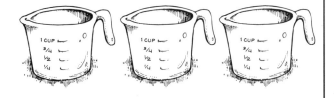

Vegetables...2 $\frac{1}{2}$ cups a day

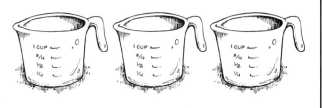

1-57029-549-2 *24-Week Health Plan*

Lessons and Activities for Week Eleven: Vegetable Stamping

Materials

Construction paper

Kitchen knife (for teacher use only)

Variety of colors of tempera paint

Shallow plates or pans

Variety of fresh vegetables

Activity

1. Remind the children how important it is to eat healthy foods. Show the children the vegetables. Challenge the children to name all of the vegetables.

2. Next, cut small pieces vegetables for the children to taste. Have them discuss which foods they prefer and which ones they need to continue tasting.

3. Cut some of the vegetables in half horizontally and some of them vertically. Fill shallow pans or plates with paint and demonstrate how to dip the vegetables into the paint and then stamp them on the paper.

4. Finally, set up an area where the children can use the vegetables to make art.

Note: Peppers cut horizontally make shamrock shapes. Tomatoes cut horizontally make interesting shapes with spots in the middle. Carrots and cucumbers cut vertically make interesting oblong shapes, while cut horizontally they make circular shapes!

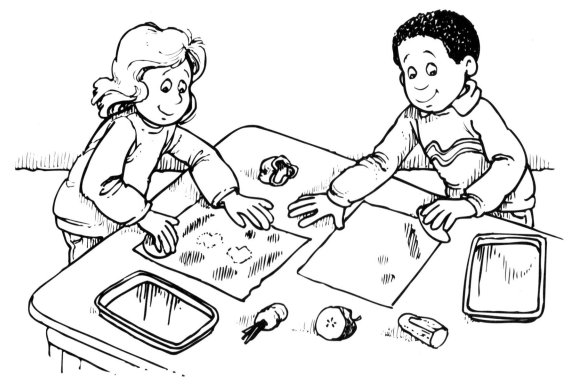

Recipe: Green Beans with Honey and Cashews

This recipe makes 20 small servings.

This recipe contains ingredients from the following food groups:

  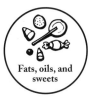

Ingredients

2 cups coarsely chopped, salted cashews

4 tablespoons unsalted butter

3 teaspoons honey

3 pounds green beans, washed and trimmed

Directions

1. Put the washed and trimmed green beans into a pot. Add water and boil the beans until they are tender-crisp. Drain and set aside.

2. In a large skillet, sauté the cashews in butter, over low heat, until they are lightly browned. This should take about five minutes.

3. Add the honey and cook, stirring constantly for one minute.

4. Pour the cashew sauce over the green beans and toss until they are coated.

Serve immediately.

 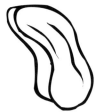 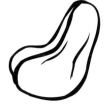

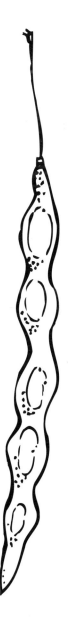

 1-57029-549-2 *24-Week Health Plan*

Exercises, Stretches, and Movement Activities

Dump Trucks Carry Vegetables

Take the children outside and demonstrate how to pretend to be a dump truck carrying a load of vegetables by bending over at the waist and holding a ball (the vegetables) on your back. Carefully "drive" around the playground. Give the children balls and have them pretend to be dump trucks carrying loads.

Then divide them into two teams. The teams should stand single-file on opposite sides of the playground. Give the first child on one of the teams a ball. The child will pretend to be a dump truck and transport the "vegetables" to the other team. The child will give the vegetables to the first person in the other team's line. This child will then pretend to be a dump truck and carry the vegetables back to the first team. The children will continue delivering back and forth until all of the children have had turns.

Transportation Vehicles Carry Vegetables

Tell the children that they will carry their "vegetables" while moving like the various transportation vehicles. Demonstrate how each vehicle will travel as follows:

- When you call out "vegetables are transported by a bicycle," the children pretend to transport vegetables by lying down on their backs and do a bicycle exercise by pretending to pedal a bicycle in the air.

- When you call out "vegetables are transported by a plane," the children pretend to transport vegetables by "flying" around the room.

- When you call out "vegetables are transported by train," the children pretend to transport vegetables by moving their arms and shuffling their feet while saying, "Choo-choo!"

- When you call out "vegetables are transported by a crane," the children pretend to transport vegetables by doing five bicep curls.

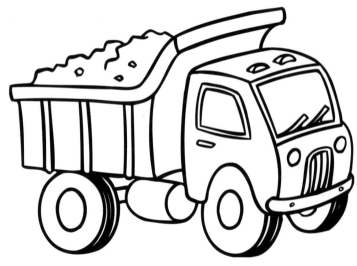

Cut the boxes apart to make a book. Staple the pages together. Draw a picture of each vegetable that you try. Color the face that shows how you feel about the new food.

I Am Trying New Vegetables!

I tasted

_____ .

I tasted

_____ .

I tasted

_____ .

I tasted

_____ .

I tasted

_____ .

1-57029-549-2 *24-Week Health Plan*

Lessons and Activities for Week Twelve: Favorite Vegetable Commercial

The children will increase vocabulary, communication, and cooperation skills as they prepare and perform a television commercial about their favorite vegetable.

Materials

Medium-sized empty cardboard box (microwave size)

Scissors

Markers

Variety of fresh or plastic vegetables

Cans of vegetables

Empty and cleaned packaging from frozen vegetables

Preparation

Make a television out of the empty cardboard box as follows:

1. Fold the top flaps inside the box.

2. Cut a large square hole in the bottom of the cardboard box.

3. Use the markers to draw details such as volume control and channel settings.

4. Make a remote control for the television. Cut a small rectangle and use the markers to draw details such as volume control and channel settings.

Lesson

1. Lead the class in a discussion about their favorite vegetables. Encourage the children to listen to their classmates' favorite vegetable selections. Explain that they will be making television commercials to advertise these favorite vegetables.

2. Have the children work together in small groups of two or three students. Encourage the small groups to decide what kind of vegetable they want to advertise. Have the children work together to create a commercial. Have the television available for the children to rehearse their commercial for several days.

3. Finally, let each group broadcast their commercial. After each commercial, give the rest of the class an opportunity to respond to the commercial by asking relevant questions or making positive statements about the commercial.

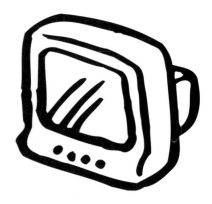

Materials

Muffin tin

Children's bag lunches

Preparation

Make a copy of the illustrated labels found at the bottom of the page. Color these labels, cut them out, and laminate. Attach them inside the muffin tin cups.

Activity

1. Review the food pyramid. Discuss why the space for grains is so much bigger than the space for oils. Point out that although all of the foods on the pyramid are important, we need more of some of the foods and less of others.

2. Have a volunteer retrieve his or her lunch box. Talk about the kinds of foods that are in the lunch box. Show the children the labeled muffin tin. Put the lunch items in the appropriate place in the muffin tin. Have the children tell if any food groups are missing. Challenge all of the children to bring in a lunch that has items from each of the food groups. Make the muffin tin available for the children to check their lunches.

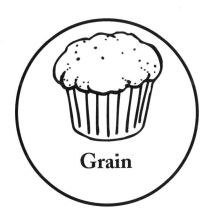
Grain

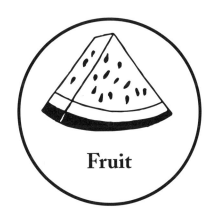
Fruit

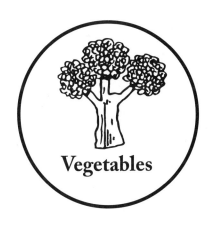
Vegetables

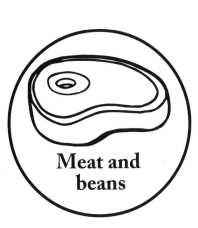
Meat and beans

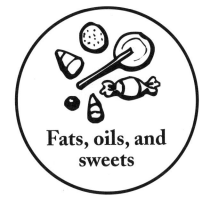
Fats, oils, and sweets

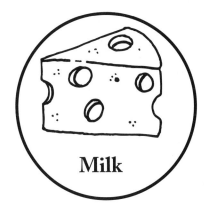
Milk

Exercises, Stretches, and Movement Activities

Race the Rolling Ball

Take the children outside and designate a "start" line and a "finish" line using chalk on a sidewalk or playground. Tell them that they are going to race against a rolling ball. Count to three and roll the ball from the starting line. The children should begin running as soon as you roll the ball. See if the ball or the children reach the finish line first!

Try rolling the ball in a variety of speeds. Start with a slow roll and increase the speed as the children get more adept at running in a group.

Roll the Dice

Show the children a pair of dice. Choose a child to name a movement activity and roll the dice, counting the dots (or adding the numbers if they are number cubes). The class will perform the movement activity named the number of times represented by the dice. For example, a child may say, "jump" and roll a five and a two on the dice. The total is equal to seven. The class will jump seven times. Other movement suggestions are:

- jump
- hop
- wiggle
- clap hands
- touch toes
- bend knees
- skip

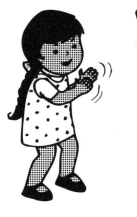 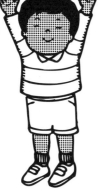 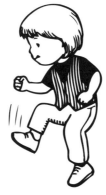

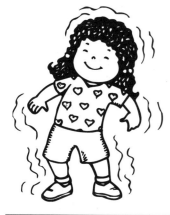 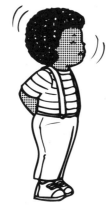 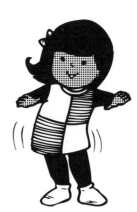 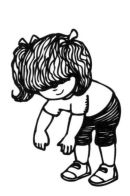 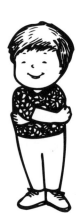

Published by Totline. Copyright protected.   1-57029-519-2 *24-Week Health Plan*

Cucumber Roll

Demonstrate how to do a cucumber roll as follows:

- Lie on the floor with your arms at your sides and your body stretched out straight like a cucumber.
- Roll in a straight line three or four times.

Have the children practice doing cucumber rolls. Encourage the children to do as many as they can without getting too dizzy.

Have the children make up other vegetable rolls for their group to do. Name them tomato rolls, potato rolls, carrot rolls, and celery stalk rolls.

Water the Vegetable Garden

The children will pretend to water the garden by standing with their arms extended straight out to the sides. They will pretend to be sprinklers by twisting their upper body towards the right and then towards the left. They will repeat this while counting to 20.

Pick the Vegetables

Have the children stretch by standing with their feet shoulder length apart. They will pretend to pick vegetables by bending at the waist and putting their hands, fingers pointing forward, flat on the ground as far in front of them as necessary for them to be able to keep their knees straight. They should breathe in and out three times, slowly, before standing up. Repeat three times.

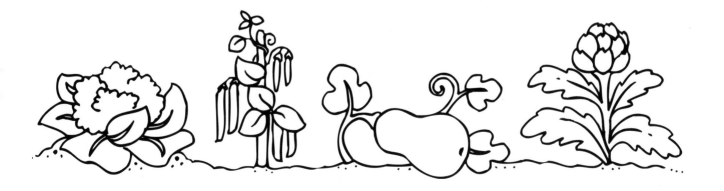

Vegetable Variety!

Directions

Fill in the blanks in each sentence. In each bowl, draw a picture of the vegetable that goes with each of your sentences.

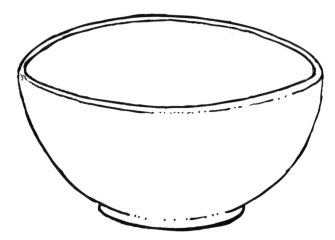

My favorite vegetable is

_____.

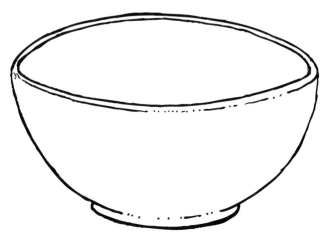

I tasted

_____

several times and still do not care for it.

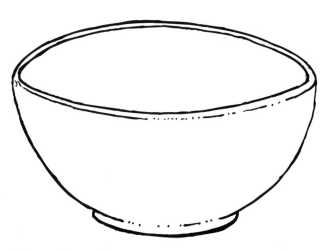

One day I want to try

_____.

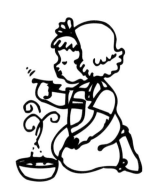

Introduction to the Fourth Month of the Health Plan

It is the start of the fourth month of *The 24-Week Health Plan*! This month children will be learning about foods from the fruit group. Children are usually more willing to try new fruit because of its natural sweetness. They will again have the opportunity to try foods and learn how to estimate correct portion sizes for the fruit group. The children will learn that fruit supplies important vitamins that help keep our gums healthy, and also help our bodies heal cuts and bruises. The children will also learn that fruit supplies us with fiber, which keeps our digestive tract healthy. The class will begin to analyze and self evaluate the fruit that they eat on a daily basis.

The children will continue participating in daily physical activity. Please incorporate the following gross motor skills into playtime:

- throwing a ball
- bouncing a ball
- catching a ball

Monthly Center

Set up an area in the classroom to serve as a fruit stand. The same set-up can be used as last month's vegetable stand. Collect a variety of fresh or plastic fruit, cans of fruit and empty and cleaned packaging from frozen fruit. Request unused foam trays or baskets from the fruit department at the local grocery store. Cut out pictures of fruit from magazines or copy and color the pictures of fruit found on page 90. Glue these pictures on to the foam trays. Include a balance scale in the center so the children can weigh the fruit. Also supply a cash register and bags so the children can pretend to buy and sell the vegetables.

Suggested activities, lessons, and games will be included in *Week Thirteen* through *Week Sixteen*. A letter to the parents, *A Tasting Diary*, *Food Tasting Rules* (just in case it is no longer hanging in the home kitchen), and *I Eat My Fruit!* should be copied and sent home to reinforce the concepts of healthy eating that are taught at school.

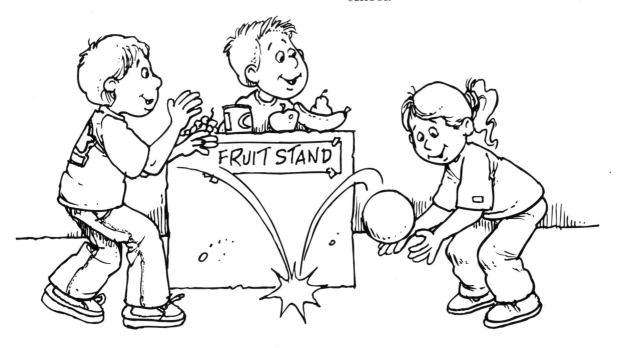

1-57029-549-2 *24-Week Health Plan*

Dear Parents:

We are beginning our fourth month of the 24-Week Health Plan! The children are becoming more willing to try a variety of new foods. Hopefully, you are having the same success at home. This month's food focus will be on fruit. Children have a much easier time incorporating fruit into their diets because of their natural sweetness. Children need at to eat at least two servings of fruit each day. Fruits help keep our gums healthy, and also help our bodies recover from cuts and bruises. Fruit also contains natural fiber, which keeps our digestive tracts healthy. Some ways to incorporate fruit into your families' diet follow:

- Breakfast: add bananas or blueberries to cereal or pancakes.
- Lunch: put grapes or applesauce into the lunchbox or mix fresh fruit with yogurt.
- Snack time: make a fruit smoothie or dip apple wedges in peanut butter or yogurt.
- Dinner: add mandarin oranges, raisins, or pear slices to salads. Serve fruit salad or strawberry shortcake for dessert.

This month, the children will continue stretching, exercising, and playing. The following gross motor skills will be incorporated into our playtime. Be sure to have your child show these to you at home.

- throwing a ball
- bouncing a ball
- catching a ball

We will also continue introducing stretches, exercises, and movement games that can be incorporated into a healthy lifestyle. Have your child teach the family some new exercises and stretches!

Have a healthy month!

Sincerely,

Materials

Newspaper

Plastic knives

Sharp knife (for adult's use only)

Watermelon

Apple

Orange

Lesson

1. Cover several tables with newspaper.

2. Read the story, *The Very Hungry Caterpillar* by Eric Carle. Lead the class in a discussion about the caterpillar's eating habits. Have the children discuss his healthy food choices and his not so healthy food choices. Also, discuss what happened when the caterpillar chooses not to eat healthy food.

3. Display the fruit that you have supplied. Have the children tell which of the fruits are their favorites. Ask the children how they could grow fruits.

4. After someone has suggested that they could plant a seed, lead the class in a discussion about where fruit seeds can be found. Tell the children that they are going to find seeds in each of the fruits that you brought. Have the children make predictions about how many seeds will be in each fruit. Write these predictions on the board or on chart paper.

5. Use the sharp knife to cut the apple and orange. Choose volunteers to help you locate and remove the seeds. Have the children count the seeds and check them against their predictions.

6. Bring the watermelon to the covered tables. Cut it open and have the children work together to remove all of the seeds. Encourage them to try the watermelon. Then have the children work together to count the seeds. Check the actual number against the children's predictions.

7. Lead the class in a discussion about which kind of fruit had the most and the least amount of seeds.

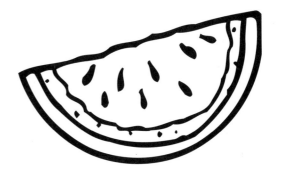

Recipe: Apple Smiles

This recipe makes one serving.

Ingredients

Two apple slices (with skin)

Peanut butter

Miniature marshmallows

Directions

1. Put one apple slice on a paper plate.

2. Spread a little bit of peanut butter on the white part of the apple. This will be the "gums."

3. Make a row of miniature marshmallows near the red skin of the apple. The marshmallows will be the "teeth."

4. Carefully put the second apple slice on top. The red skin of the apples makes the lips and now you have a beautiful smile!

Note: These smiles can be customized to suit the child. If a child is missing a front tooth, remove one of his or her marshmallows.

This recipe contains ingredients from the following food groups:

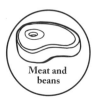

Meat and beans

Fruit

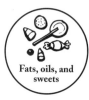

Fats, oils, and sweets

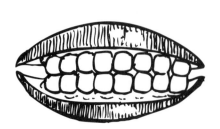

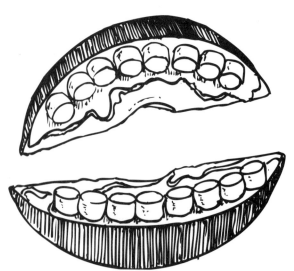

1-57029-519-2   *24-Week Health Plan*

Pick the Apples!

Have the children stretch up and pretend to reach high to pick apples from a tree. Teach the children the following poem:

Pick the Apples!

I reach up high with my arms,

When I'm at the apple farm.

On my tiptoes, I do stand,

To reach the apples with my hand.

I grab it then I give a pull.

And eat the apple 'til I'm full!

Have the children repeat the poem as they pretend to pick apples. Challenge the children to stay on their tiptoes for longer stretches of time each time they say the poem.

Walking/Running on TipToes

Take the children outside and have them walk across the basketball court or playground on their tiptoes. Then challenge the children to run on their tiptoes over the same course.

Calf Stretches

Before and after running activities as well as the two activities listed above, it is important to have the children warm up their muscles first. Teach the children to stretch their calf muscles as follows:

- Stand up and place both hands on a wall.
- Step backwards with your right foot, so that only your toes are touching the floor.
- Bend your left knee and try to touch your right heel to the ground.
- Count to five.
- Switch feet.
- Repeat this three times.

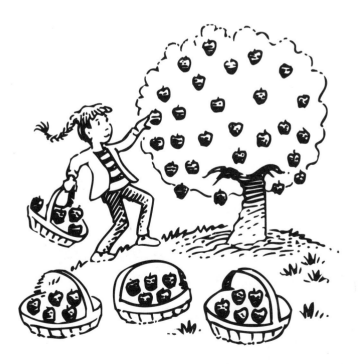

Are You Eating Enough Fruit?

It is easy to eat enough fruit every day. Just have a little fruit with each meal!

In the morning, I can eat a

_____ with my breakfast.

I like to eat

_____ with my lunch.

In the afternoon, I like to eat

_____ for a snack.

At night, I can eat

_____ with my
dinner.

Lessons and Activities for Week Fourteen: Favorite Fruit Graph

Materials

Chart paper or poster board

Markers

Crayons

Activity

1. Divide a large poster board or chart into six columns.

2. Read a story about fruit to the class. Have the children tell about their favorite parts the book.

3. Then, have the children brainstorm a list of fruit. Choose six of the fruits that the children named. Write one fruit at the bottom of each column of your graph.

4. Explain that you are interested in finding out how many children like the fruit listed on the graph. Explain that you are curious about which of these fruits will be the class "favorite." Give each child an opportunity to tell which is his or her favorite. Have the children write their names in the column above their favorite fruits. When all of the children have had a chance to participate, have the children count the names in each column and write the totals at the top.

Then lead the class in a discussion about the results of the graph. Some sample questions follow:

- How many children like (name one of the fruits from the graph)?

- How many children like (name another fruit from the graph)?

- Which fruit is the most popular? How can you tell?

- Which fruit is the least popular? How can you tell?

5. Display the graph in the classroom. Suggest that it might be fun for the children to make their own graphs and interview their friends about food during free time.

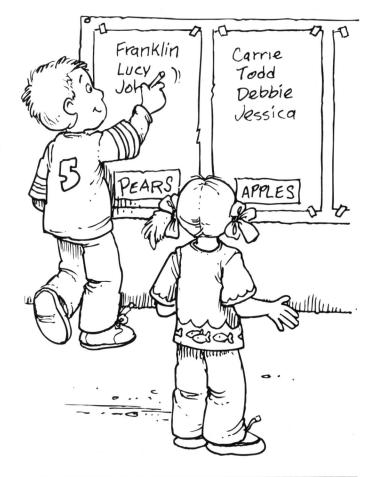

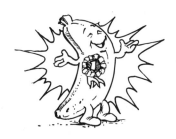

Recipe: Cooperative Fruit Salad

The children will work together to clean and cut fruit for a fresh fruit salad.

Materials

Plastic knives

Large bowl

Unusual fruits such as coconut, star fruit, kiwi

Activity

1. Lead the class in a discussion about the fun of working together to make a snack. Then discuss what it would be like if everyone brought in a different piece of fruit, washed them, cut them up, and put it in a bowl to make fruit salad for everyone to share.

2. Make a copy of one grocery list (found at the bottom of the page) for each child to take home. Have each child dictate the name of his or her favorite fruit. Then have each child illustrate and take home his or her list.

3. When the children bring their fruit to school, have them count the fruit and work together to classify the fruit by kind, size, or color. Be sure to include the unusual fruit that you supplied. Next, have the children work together to wash, cut, and assemble the fruit salad.

4. While everyone is enjoying the fruit salad, encourage the children to try new fruit and discuss the benefit of having everyone bring fruit to school.

Grocery List	**Grocery List**	**Grocery List**
I want to bring	I want to bring	I want to bring
_____	_____	_____
for our fruit salad.	for our fruit salad.	for our fruit salad.

Exercises, Stretches, and Movement Activities

The Three Little Pigs

Your "little pigs" will enjoy and benefit from this running activity as it encourages a deep breathing break following short running bursts (cardio workouts).

Set up three areas that will represent the three houses in the story *The Three Little Pigs*. These houses should be separated by a distance that the children can comfortably run.

Before the "little pigs" begin, have them stretch their legs and arms. Then demonstrate deep breathing as follows:

Take three slow, deep breaths, nodding your head three times during the intake of air and nodding your head three times as they let the air out.

Have the children practice taking slow, deep breaths. Then have them run to the first house and stop. Take three slow, deep breaths. After breathing, have them run to the second house and then stop to breathe again. Finally, they will run to the third house and stop to breathe again.

Note: Make sure the children know that they should breathe regularly while they run!

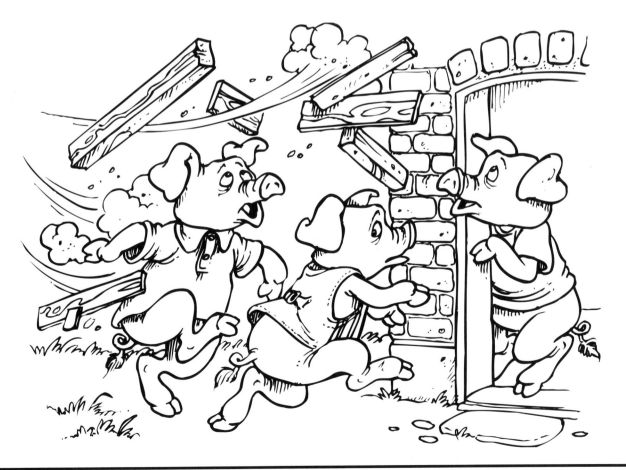

I Eat My Fruit!

Directions

Draw the fruit you eat each day, for the next four days. Remember to eat at least two servings of fruit each day!

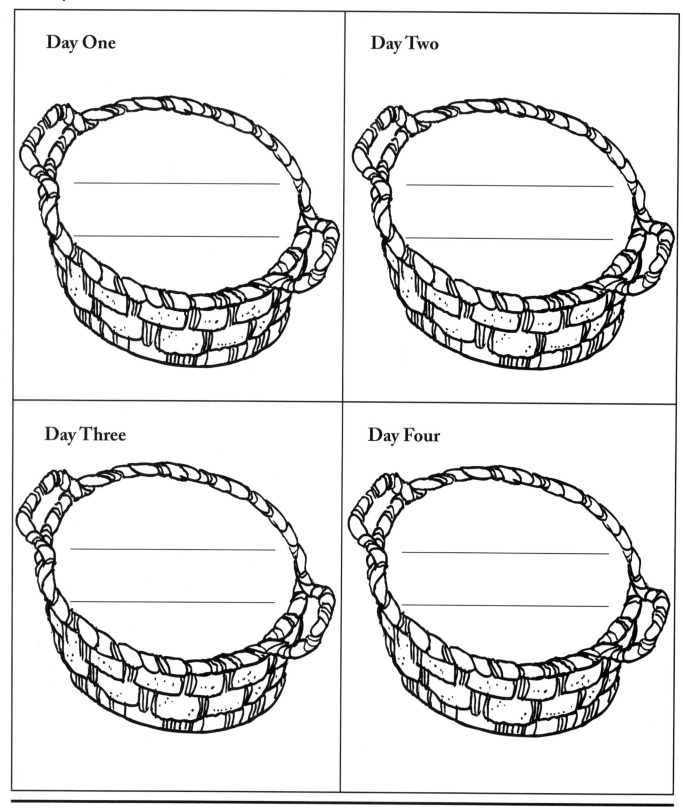

Day One

Day Two

Day Three

Day Four

1-57029-519-2 *24-Week Health Plan*

Materials

Variety of fruit (banana, watermelon, apple, orange, strawberry, kiwi, grape)

Shallow tub

Water

One copy of page 88 for each child

Preparation

Fill up the tub with water and set up an area where the children can test the various fruit to see if they sink or float.

Activity

1. Show the children the fruit that you brought to school. Ask them to name the fruit and tell whether or not they have ever tried them.

2. Ask the children what they know about things that sink and things that float.

3. Tell the children that they will be performing an experiment to find out which kinds of fruit sink and which kinds float. Show the children the fruit. Have the children make predictions. Write their predictions on the board or on chart paper. Point out that it is not important to make "correct" predictions. Explain that predictions get your brain ready to think about the scientific outcomes of the experiment.

4. Allow all of the children an opportunity to "test" the fruit.

5. When all of the children have had a chance to perform the experiment, lead the class in a discussion about the results. Discuss which fruit floated. Have the children come up with ideas as to why these fruits floated. Then discuss the fruits that sunk.

6. Finally, wash and cut the fruit. Give the children an opportunity to taste the different kinds.

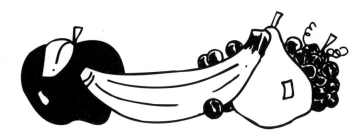

Some Fruits Sink and Some Fruits Float

Draw the fruits that float at the top of the water. Draw the fruits that sink underneath the waterline.

How many fruits floated?_____

How many fruits sunk?_____

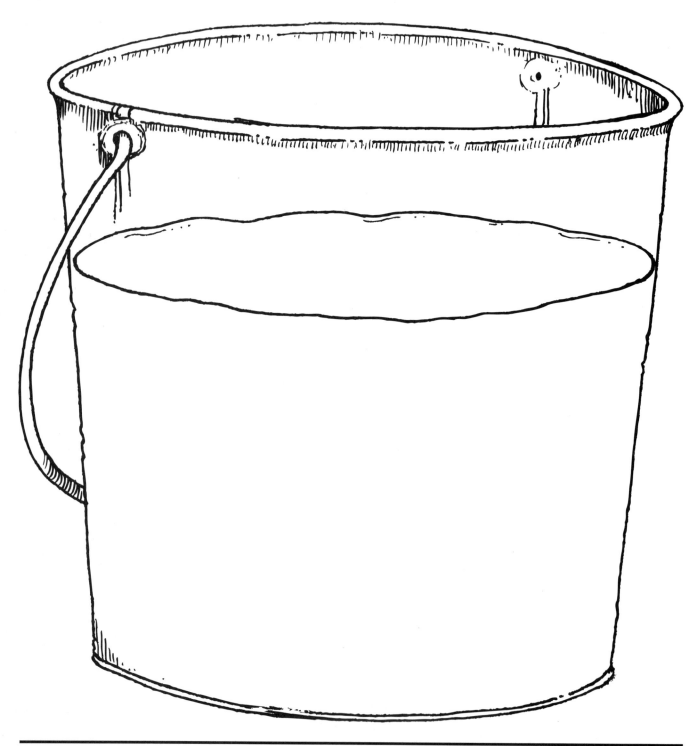

Food Pyramid Activity: We're Going on a Picnic

Materials

Real and plastic food items, including pictures of food (laminate for durability)

Directions

1. Tell the children that they are going on a pretend picnic. Explain that each child will bring a food item.

2. Have the children sit in a circle on the floor and put all of the food items in the middle of the circle.

3. Demonstrate how to play as follows:

   - Say, "We are going on a picnic and I am going to bring a (example: banana). My banana is from the fruit group." Then take a real, plastic, or photo of a banana from the middle of the circle.

   - Have the child sitting to your left do the same as you. He or she will say, "We are going on a picnic and my teacher is bringing a banana from the fruit group and I am bringing (example: bread) from the grain group."

   - The game gets harder as it progresses!

   - Continue playing in this manner until all of the children have selected an item and named everyone else's choices.

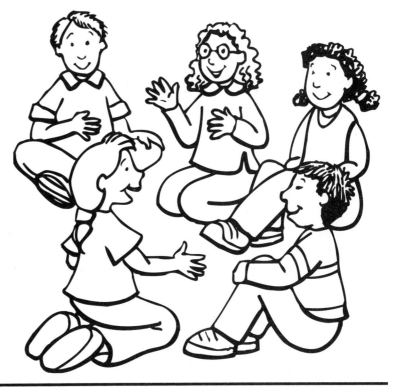

Exercises, Stretches, and Movement Activities

Balance

Tell the children that in some countries, people balance baskets on their heads when they go to the market to buy fruit. They fill the baskets with their fruit and walk back home. Make a "balance beam" on the carpet with duct tape or use chalk outside on the sidewalk. Have the children take turns strengthening their balancing skills by traveling, with pretend fruit baskets on their heads, across the balance beam. They can walk, hop, tiptoe, or move in any way across the beam.

Star Fruit Stretch

For this stretch, the children will lie on their backs with their arms and legs comfortably stretched out. They will raise their right arms towards the ceiling and then lower them. Children repeat this with their left arms. Then, they will lift the right legs towards the ceiling and then lower them. They will repeat this with their left legs. Finally, they will try lifting one arm and the opposite leg at the same time and lower them. They will repeat this with the opposite arms and legs. Repeat these stretches three times.

This stretch helps to increase the flexibility and coordination of the arms and legs.

The Banana Peel Stretch

Pretend you are a banana. Lie on the floor on your back. Now, someone is going to peel you. Pull one of your knees towards your chest. Hug your knee and count to five. Repeat with the other leg (the other side of the peel!). This stretches your back.

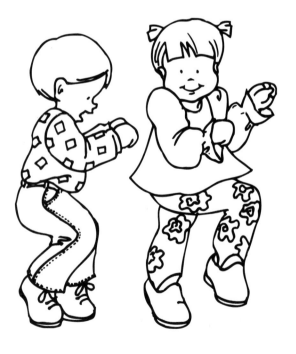

Published by Totline. Copyright protected.   1-57029-519-2   *24-Week Health Plan*

Lessons and Activities for Week Sixteen: Fabulous Fruit!

Materials

Chart paper

Variety of fruit (real, plastic, pictures, containers, or cans)

Directions

1. Lead the class in a discussion about their favorite kinds of fruit. List the children's favorite fruit on the board or on chart paper.

2. Suggest the children sort the fruit according to color. Designate areas on a tabletop for each color of fruit. Have one child at a time choose a fruit and put it into the appropriate spot.

3. After all the children have sorted the fruit by color, take a class survey. Write each fruit color group on the board or on chart paper. Ask the children the following question:

   • What color group is your favorite fruit in?

4. Have the children raise their hands as you call out each color or sign their names underneath the color group of their choice.

5. Finally, lead the class in a discussion about the results of both the graph and the survey. Some sample questions for discussion follow:

   • Which color group contains the most fruit?

   • Which color group contains the least fruit?

   • How many more pieces of fruit are in the group with the most than the group with the least?

   • Which color fruit is the most popular with the class?

   • Which color fruit is the least popular with the class?

Finally, point out how important it is to eat a variety of fruit since different fruit helps keep our bodies healthy in different ways.

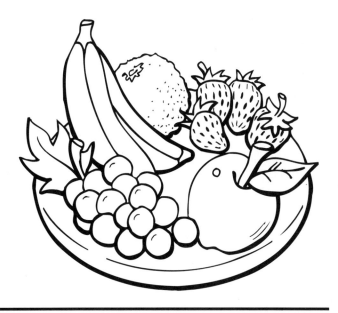

 1-57029-549-2 *24-Week Health Plan*

Food Pyramid Lesson: Guess My Food!

Materials

Five craft sticks

Orange, green, red, blue, and purple markers

Cup or can

Preparations

Color each craft stick a different color.

Lesson

1. Review the food groups. Have the children name foods from each group. Tell the children that they will be playing a game. They will try to guess what food their friends are thinking of.

2. Show the children the cup of colored craft sticks. Explain that each colored stick will represent one of the food groups in the food pyramid. Tell the children which color each stick will represent. Make a chart, or write the list on the board.

   • Orange—Grain group

   • Green—Vegetable group

   • Red—Fruit group

   • Blue—Milk group

   • Purple—Meat and bean group

3. Have a volunteer choose a stick from the cup. Have the child whisper a food that comes from the food group chosen. Then have the child begin giving out hints to the class about his or her food choice. For example, a child chooses an orange stick. He chooses the food spaghetti and whispers this in his teacher's ear. Then he gives out the following clues:

   • It is served hot.

   • It is yellowish-tan.

   • It is served with red sauce.

   • It is wiggly.

   • You might like meatballs with this.

4. You might want to stretch this activity over several days, only allowing three or four children to participate each day.

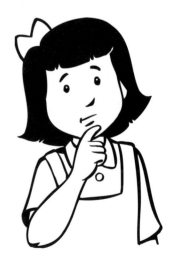

Bounce to the Beat

Bring large playground balls outside and have the children practice their ball bouncing skills. Have the children drop the ball from hip level and try to catch it as it bounces up. More advanced children can lightly toss the ball up and catch it. As the children improve their ball bouncing skills, encourage them to try to bounce the ball to the steady beat of slow music.

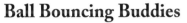

Ball Bouncing Buddies

Have the children pair up. Have them practice bouncing a ball to their partner. The partner will then try to catch the ball as it bounces and return it with a bounce. For advanced children, have them stand further away from each other. You can also use different sized balls for a challenge. The bouncing will have to be more accurately aimed.

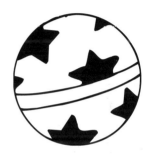

Catch!

Take beach balls outside. Lightly toss the beach ball to the children and have the children practice catching them. Beach balls work well for beginners because they are less likely to hurt a child if he or she is hit in the face when trying to catch the ball! Pair the children up and have them practice throwing and catching the beach balls. Have the children stand close together because the beach balls are light, making them hard to throw far distances.

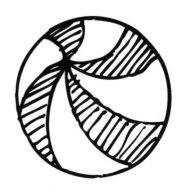

Fresh Fruit Patterns

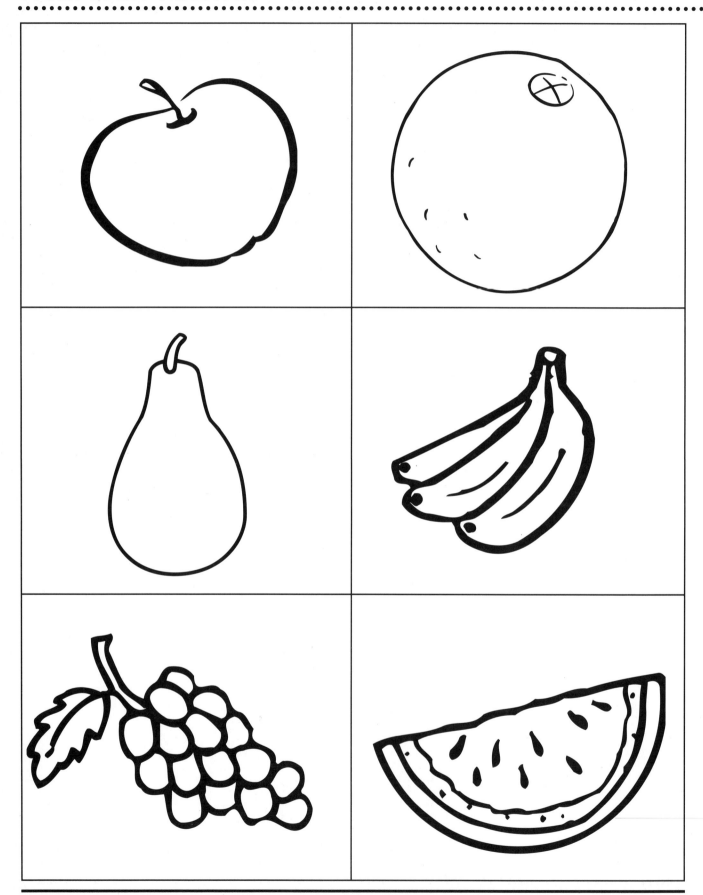

This month the children will be learning the importance of including foods from the milk group in their daily diet. They will be learning about the different foods that are made from milk and will also learn how the calcium in milk products helps keep our bones and teeth healthy and strong. The children will learn to analyze and self-evaluate the milk products that they eat on a daily basis.

The children will continue participating in daily physical activity. The children will recognize the importance of daily stretching, exercising, and gross motor movement. Incorporate the following gross motor skills into playtime:

- jumping over low obstacles
- running, hopping, and galloping around obstacles

Monthly Center

Set up an area in the classroom to serve as an old-fashioned ice cream parlor to stimulate the children's creativity during free time. Include a variety of cups and bowls in different sizes, ice cream scoops, disposable straws, plastic fruit, cookie cutters, and plastic spoons. Purchase or make modeling dough to include in the center. The dough can be colored and scented so that children can pretend it is ice cream, or make pieces of fruit and other toppings

Suggested activities, lessons, and games will be included in *Week Seventeen* through *Week Twenty*. A letter to the parents, *A Tasting Diary*, and *Mighty Milk Products* should be copied and sent home to reinforce the concepts about dairy products that will be introduced at school.

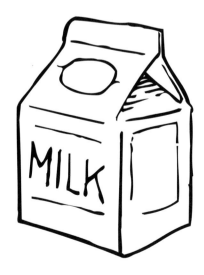

Dear Parents:

We are beginning our fifth month of the 24-Week Health Plan! The children are learning a lot about healthy choices, both with the foods they eat and with the physical activities they participate in. This month the children will begin to document how much time they spend "playing" and compare it to how much time they spend watching television and playing video games. The children will continue stretching, exercising, and playing in physically active games. The following gross motor skills will be incorporated into our playtime. Encourage your child to practice these gross motor skills at home, too.

- jumping over low obstacles
- running, hopping, and galloping around obstacles

We will be making obstacle courses at school. The children will no doubt enjoy creating their own obstacle courses at home for their families and friends to "work out" with.

This month the children will be learning about food from the milk group. They will learn that many of the foods that they enjoy eating each day are made from milk. Children, ages two years to eight years, should have at least two cups of milk products each day. This can include milk, yogurt, cheese, cottage cheese, ice cream, and more. The children will make homemade butter and ice cream so they can see first hand how milk is part of these foods.

Please let us know how your child is incorporating healthy food and exercise choices in his or her home life!

Have a healthy month!

Sincerely,

Lessons and Activities for Week Seventeen: Milk Moustaches

Materials

Milk

Paper cups

Camera with film

Construction paper

Markers

Crayons

Activity

1. Lead the class in a discussion about what they know about how milk is "made." Then read a book about milk to the class. *Milk: From Cow to Carton* by Aliki and *The Milk Makers* by Gail Gibbons are good illustrations of how we get milk. Have the children tell about their favorite parts of the book.

2. Explain that milk and milk products are important because they contain calcium. Calcium is important because it helps make our bones and teeth healthy and strong.

3. Give each child a glass of milk. Take a picture of each child wearing his or her "milk moustache."

4. Have the class work together to make a book, titled "Our Milk Moustaches!" Each child will complete the following sentence prompt:

   I drink milk because it helps me

   _____.

   Each child will illustrate his or her sentence on a separate sheet of art paper.

5. Have the film developed and then glue each child's photograph to his or her page. After binding the book, read it to the class and store it in the classroom library.

Optional

These pages also make a cute bulletin board display!

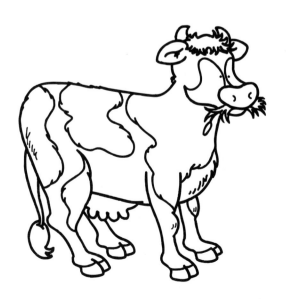

Recipe: Smoothies

This recipe makes two small smoothies.

Ingredients

1 cup milk

Fresh or frozen fruit (strawberries, blueberries, bananas, or combination)

Ice

Wax paper (optional)

Directions

Cut the fruit into chunks. Put all ingredients into a blender and blend until smooth. Serve.

Tip: The night before, peel the bananas, cut them into thirds, lay them on wax paper, and freeze them. The frozen bananas give the smoothie an "ice cream" texture.

This recipe contains ingredients from the following food groups:

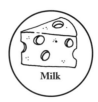

Milk

Fruit

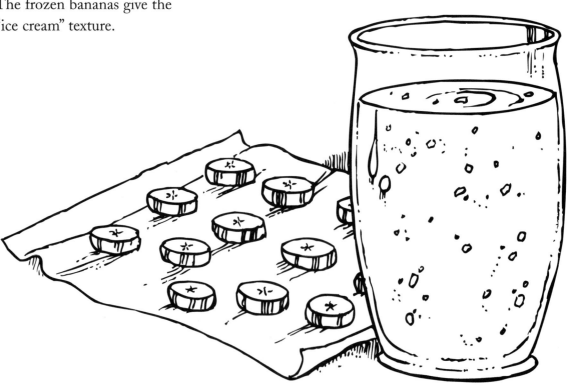

Exercises, Stretches, and Movement Activities

Low Limbo

Make a "low limbo" by laying a jump rope in a straight line on the floor. Have the children take turns jumping over it. Then have a volunteer help you make the "low limbo" a little bit higher by stretching a jump rope and holding it two inches above the ground. Again, have the children take turns jumping over the "low limbo." Continue to raise the "low limbo" as the children become comfortable, but do not raise it higher than six inches above the ground.

A more challenging low limbo could involve having the children hop over the rope on one foot or hopping over and then immediately back. Having the children wiggle over like a piece of spaghetti or jump over like a bean could also be fun!

Obstacle Course

Set up an obstacle course in the classroom or outside. When the children reach an obstacle, they will jump over it, run around it, or crawl under it. Before beginning the obstacle course, explain your expectations as to what the children will do when they reach each obstacle. Choose a volunteer to demonstrate how to move through the obstacle course. Allow the children to move though the course several times. They will increase their coordination and speed ability with practice.

Be sure to set realistic goals for the height of obstacles or the length of the run or hopping that they will have to do. While some children are very coordinated others are still developing the gross motor skills necessary to accomplish the course.

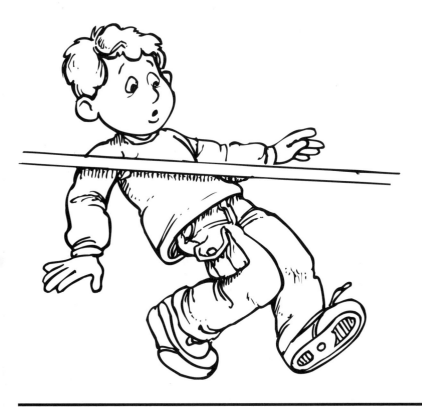

Delicious Dairy Patterns

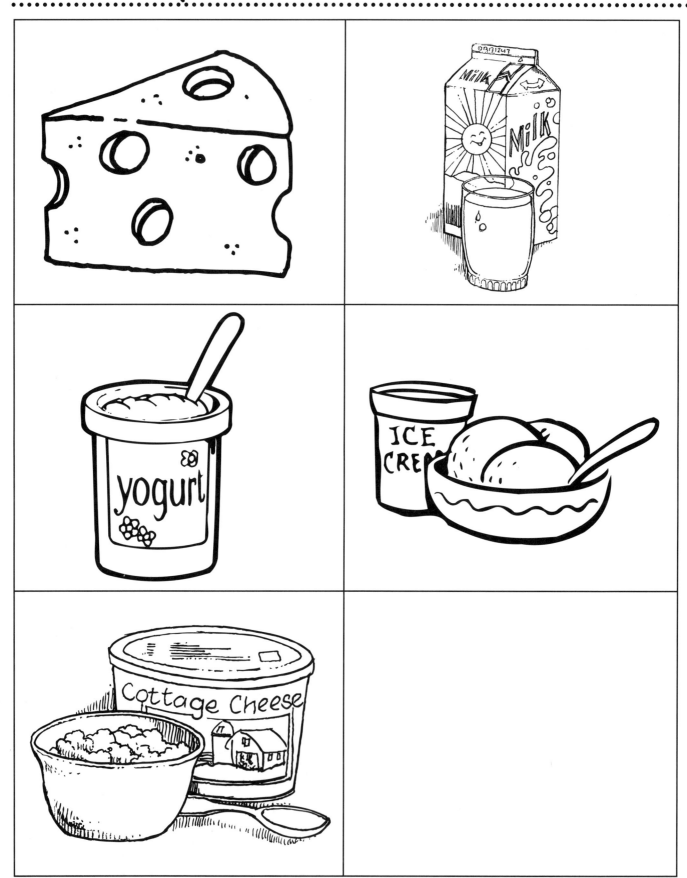

Materials

Real and plastic food items

Pictures of food (If using the food patterns from this book cut, color, and laminate for durability.)

Lesson

1. Have the children answer the following questions:

   • Do you want to grow up tall and strong?

   • Do you want to have a lot of energy for school and play?

   • Do you want to be healthy?

   Explain that if they answered "Yes!" to the above questions, then they need to eat a variety of foods from the five food groups every day.

2. Teach the children the following cheer. Have each child choose a favorite food to hold up at the end when they say, "Yeah!"

Yeah!

Yes, yes, yes! We want to be strong.

So we eat healthy all day long!

We eat fruit and veggies, too.

We eat meat and grain, do you?

We love to drink our milk each day.

Now we have energy to play!

Yeah!

Note

This is a good cheer to say before lunch as it encourages them to make healthy food choices! Also, say it before recess as it reinforces the fact that healthy food gives them energy they need to play!

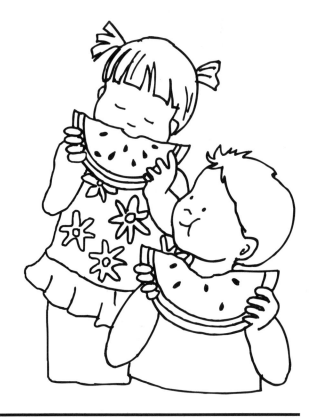

Recipe: Cheesy Cider Fondue

Ingredients

4 cups (1 pound) shredded Cheddar cheese

$2\frac{1}{2}$ teaspoons cornstarch

$1\frac{1}{4}$ cups apple cider

$\frac{1}{2}$ cup lemon juice

$\frac{1}{2}$ teaspoon salt

$\frac{1}{8}$ teaspoon cinnamon

$\frac{1}{8}$ teaspoon nutmeg

Freshly ground pepper

For dipping

Bite-size pieces of cooked chicken or pork sausages

Grapes

French bread, cut into cubes

Apple wedges

Pretzels

Directions

1. In a medium-size bowl, toss the cheese and cornstarch.

2. In a medium-size, heavy-bottomed saucepan, heat the cider and lemon juice over medium heat until it is simmering.

3. Add the cheese, one handful at a time. Stir the mixture until each handful of cheese is melted before adding more.

4. When all the cheese has been added, stir in the salt, cinnamon, nutmeg, and pepper.

5. Cook over low heat until the cheese mixture has thickened. This will take about 3 to 5 minutes.

6. Pour into a bowl and serve immediately.

This recipe contains ingredients from the following food groups:

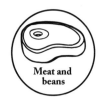
Meat and beans

Fruit

Milk

Grain

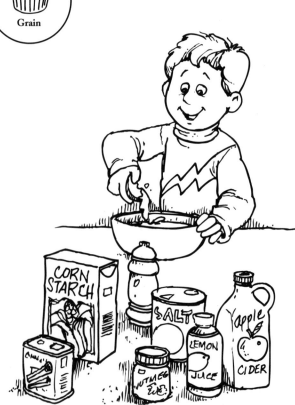

1-57029-519-2 *24-Week Health Plan*

Even characters in stories depend on stretching to keep themselves flexible and healthy. With all of the running around and crazy situations they find themselves in, it is a good thing they remember to stretch out first!

Goldilocks' Wake Up Stretch

Pretend that you are just waking up. Stretch your arms as high up to the sky as you can. Hold this stretch for five seconds. Now reach up higher with your right hand, then the left. Alternate like this for ten counts.

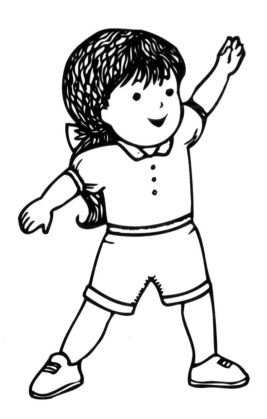

The Wolf Takes Deep Cleansing Breaths

Before the wolf goes out to catch the pigs or Little Red Riding Hood, he relaxes by taking deep, cleansing breaths. This also helps him calm down when he is feeling angry! Try it next time you feel upset.

Have the children sit down on the floor, with their knees bent and the soles of their feet touching. Have them slowly take in a deep breath through their noses and hold it for three counts. Then have them let the air out slowly through their mouths, making the phonetic S sound. (They should sound like a tire with air leaking out.) Repeat this five times.

Now that you have warmed up try this *Little Red Hen* activity!

The Little Red Hen

Have the children be cooperative participants in this story rather than the lazy ones depicted in the original story. Have the children move around while they pretend to plow the field, plant the wheat seeds, pull the weeds, cut the wheat, carry it to the mill. Next, encourage the children to carry out the little red hen's chores in "fast motion."

Recipe: Butter

Ingredients

1 pint heavy cream

salt (optional)

crackers

Other Materials

Jar with a tight fitting lid (at least quart sized)

Several marbles

Plates

Plastic knives

Directions

1. Pour the cream into the jar.

2. Add salt to taste (just a shake or two will do).

3. Put the marbles into the cream. The marbles will aid in the shaking process.

4. Close the jar, making sure the seal is tight. Shake, shake, and shake! Let each child have a turn shaking!

5. The cream will become whipping cream first. Then the cream will begin to solidify. Continue shaking until you see a solid mass of butter. The liquid part is buttermilk!

6. Pour the buttermilk off. Remove all of the marbles and have the children spread the butter on crackers.

Enjoy!

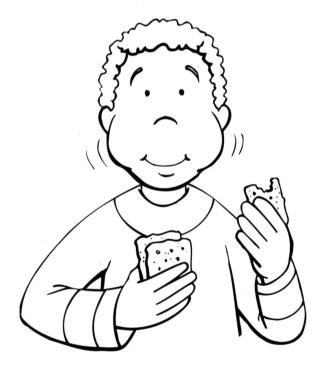

Lessons and Activities for Week Nineteen: Painting Pita Bread

Materials

Several different kinds of yogurt in a variety of colors

Clean paintbrushes

Pita bread

Plates

Lesson

1. Read the children a book about products derived from milk. (Some suggestions are found in the main booklist.) Discuss how many different kinds of foods that they regularly enjoy are made from milk. Have the children name some of these foods (yogurt, cheese, butter, ice cream).

2. Explain that they will be creating an edible work of art using yogurt as "paint" and pita bread as the "canvas." Demonstrate how to dip a paintbrush into the yogurt and "paint" on the pita bread.

3. After the children have created masterpieces, let them have a snack!

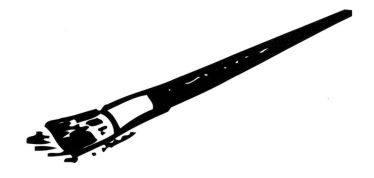

Recipe: Apple Pie Through a Straw

Makes one *Apple Pie Through a Straw* drink.

Ingredients

1 cup low fat milk

$\frac{1}{2}$ cup apple sauce

$\frac{1}{2}$ teaspoon cinnamon

$1\frac{1}{2}$ teaspoons sugar

Additional Supplies

Measuring cup

One straw and cup for each child

One shaking container with a tight fitting lid
or a blender

Directions

Measure the ingredients and put them all in the
"shaking container" or blender. Shake or blend
well. Pour the drink in a glass and enjoy!

This recipe contains ingredients from the
following food groups:

 Milk

 Fruit

 Fats, oils, and sweets

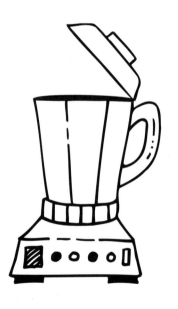

The children will demonstrate and increase their flexibility as they create shapes with their bodies during stretching.

Triangle Stretch

The children will begin this stretch by sitting on the floor with their legs straight out in front of them. They will stretch their arms straight up over their heads and then reach down to touch their toes, keeping their knees as straight as possible. They will hold their bodies in the shape of a triangle for five seconds. Repeat this three times.

Circle Stretch

The children will begin this stretch lying flat on the floor. They will pull their knees into their chests and wrap their arms around their knees and squeeze tightly. Hold this stretch for a count of five. Repeat this three times.

Angle Stretch

The children will begin this stretch sitting on the floor with their legs open in a "V" position. They lean their bodies down towards their left leg, trying to reach their left toes with both hands and touch their noses to their knees. They will hold this stretch for five seconds. Then they will switch sides and stretch towards their right leg, trying to reach their right toes with both hands and touch their noses to their knees. They will hold this stretch for five seconds. Repeat three times.

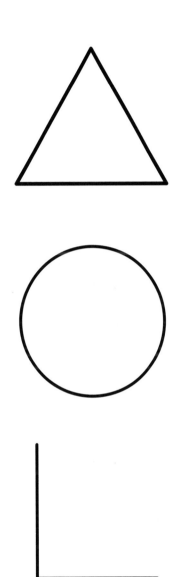

Recipe: Ice Cream in a Bag

Ingredients

1 tablespoon granulated sugar

$\frac{1}{2}$ cup milk or half-and-half

$\frac{1}{4}$ teaspoon vanilla extract

6 tablespoons rock salt

Other Supplies

1 pint-size zip-type plastic bag

1 gallon-size zip-type plastic bag

Directions

1. Fill the large bag half full of ice, and add the rock salt. Seal the bag.

2. Put milk, vanilla extract, and sugar into the small bag, and seal it.

3. Open the large bag and place the small bag inside the large one. Seal the large one again.

4. Shake until mixture is ice cream, about five minutes.

5. Wipe off top of small bag, then open carefully and enjoy!

This recipe contains ingredients from the following food groups:

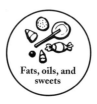

Fats, oils, and sweets

Milk

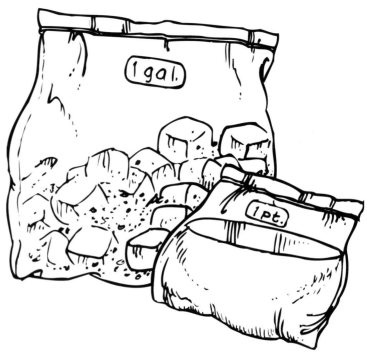

Directions:

Keep track of how many milk products you have each day. Color one glass of milk for each dairy serving you enjoy! Children ages two to eight should have two cups of dairy products each day. Children older than eight should have three cups of dairy products each day.

Monday	Tuesday	Wednesday	Thursday	Friday

Milk Lotto Game

This game is to be played with a group of two to four children.

Preparation

Copy the lotto cards found on page 111 onto tag board, making enough for four children. Make three copies of the matching cards below. Cut out these cards. Laminate the lotto cards and the matching cards for durability.

How to Play

Stack the matching cards facedown on the table. Give each child a lotto card. Have the first child draw one matching card from the pile. If it matches a picture on the child's card, he or she will place the picture on top of the matching picture on his lotto card. If it does not, the child will discard the picture. The next child will either choose the discarded picture or draw a card from the pile and see if it matches his or her card. The play continues in this manner until one of the children matches all of the pictures on his or her card.

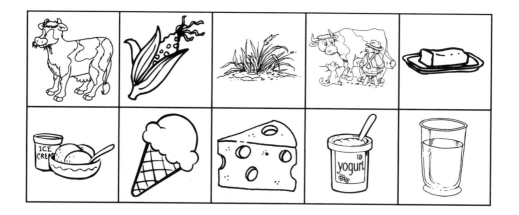

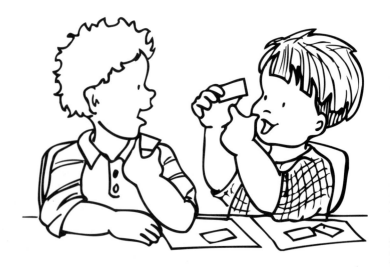

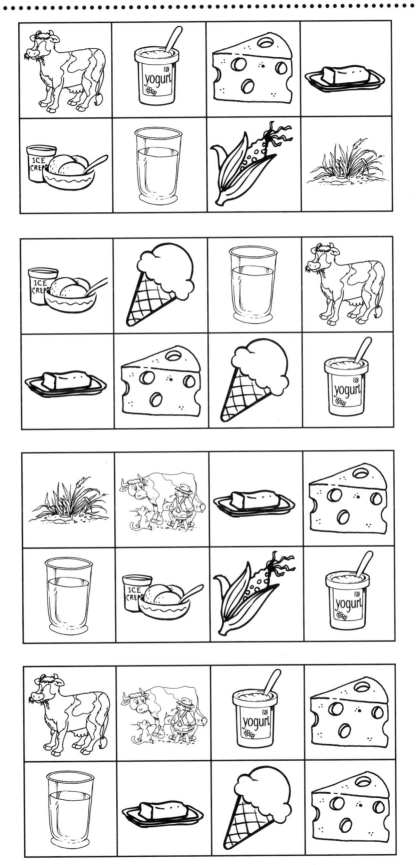

1-57029-549-2 *24-Week Health Plan*

Birds at Home!

This is an outside game to be played in an open space. Divide the children into groups of three. Have two of the children form the "house" by standing face-to-face while raising their arms and touching their fingers. The third child will be the "bird" who lives in the "house." When you call out, "Fly, birds, fly!" the birds will run around and look for new houses. Then the runner will change places with one of the house people and the house person will become a bird. Every time you call "Fly, birds, fly!" the children will run to different houses. When you call out, "Home, Tweet, Home!" the children will have to run and find their original partners, making a house for their original bird.

Leapfrog

This is an old game that allows the children to practice cooperation skills while increasing their upper and lower body strength.

Divide the children into pairs. Have the first child squat down. The second child will put his or her hands on top of the first child's back. He or she will then leap over the child's back and squat down in front. The squatting child will then stand up, put his or her hands on the squatting child's back and leap over. The children will continue working together in this way as they travel across the classroom or an open field.

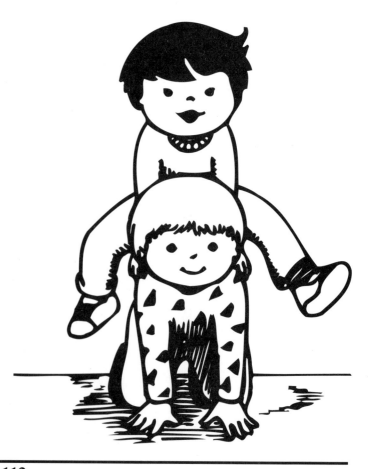

Introduction to the Sixth Month of the Health Plan

Welcome to the last month of *The 24-Week Health Plan*. Hopefully the children are incorporating healthy foods into their diets as well as participating in daily physical play! The children will learn about the different types of protein and also continue to analyze and self-evaluate the meals that they eat on a daily basis, making sure to include enough protein.

Take care when discussing the original source of meat proteins. Some young children may become upset when they learn that their favorite meats were once living pigs, cows, or lambs. Often when children visualize animals, they think of animals seen in children's books or movies. Not only are these animals cute and cuddly, but they are usually personified. Also, keep in mind that some children in the class may be vegetarians. These children do not eat meat at all. A vegetarian meets his or her daily protein requirement by eating whole grains, nuts, seeds, beans, dairy, and vegetables. If any of the children in the class are vegetarian, invite the family to prepare a vegetarian meal for the class.

The children should now recognize the importance of daily stretching, exercising, and gross motor movement to overall good health. Incorporate the following skills during playtime:

- jumping over several low objects in a row

- skipping

- walking forward and backward in a straight line heel-to-toe

Monthly Center

Set up an area to serve as a meat department. Collect a variety of non-perishable protein items (cans of nuts, tuna fish, clams, chicken). The meat department can also be stocked with clean, unused foam meat trays with pictures of different kinds of meat glued to the trays. Include a scale. You can make the foam trays different weights by taping different amounts of pennies underneath the pictures of meat.

Suggested activities, lessons, and games are included in *Week Twenty One* through *Week Twenty Four*. A letter to the parents, *Healthy Chicken Nuggets*, *A Tasting Diary*, *TV Verses Playtime*, *Protein Delivers a Powerful Punch!*, and *What Do I Eat?* should all be copied and sent home to reinforce the concepts about healthy food choices and physical activities.

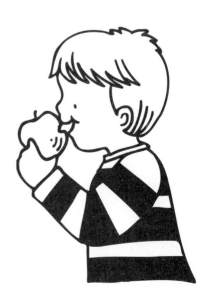

Dear Parents,

We are beginning our last month of the 24-Week Health Plan! The children have learned a lot about healthy choices, both with the foods they eat and with the physical activities they participate in. The following gross motor skills will be incorporated into our playtime. Be sure to do these with your child at home.

- jumping over several low objects in a row

- skipping

- walking forward and backward in a straight line heel-to-toe

This month we will be learning about the importance of eating protein. It is an extremely important nutrient because it builds muscles and bones and provides us with needed energy. Protein can also help with weight control because protein helps you feel full and satisfied from your meals for a longer period of time.

Very often the main source of protein for children is the popular chicken nugget. The chicken nugget is really junk food disguised as a healthy choice of protein. Here are some facts about chicken nuggets:

- 50% to 60% of the calories in most nuggets come from fat.

- Chicken nuggets are highly processed. Highly processed food is one of the main reasons the percentage of overweight kids has tripled in the past 20 years! Many nuggets are made of a combination of meat and chicken skin.

  The chicken parts are ground into small bits and binders are added to make the "chicken" stick together. Then it is pressed into the traditional nugget shape. The nugget is then deep fried in hydrogenated oil. Most nuggets have more grams of fat and carbohydrates than grams of protein!

- There are some chicken nuggets that contain all white meat, however, the label needs to say "all-white meat" for this to be true. A Healthy Chicken Nugget recipe will be prepared in class and a copy of this will also be sent home.

Please let us know how your child is incorporating healthy food and exercise choices in his or her home life! Also, if you have any interesting recipes or suggestions to encourage healthy eating or exercise, please share them with us!

Thank you for all of your support and continue to have healthy months!

Sincerely,

Materials

Two copies of the Protein Playing Cards
(page 116)

Tag board

Crayons

Scissors

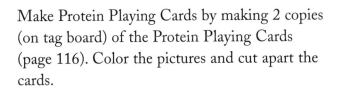

Make Protein Playing Cards by making 2 copies
(on tag board) of the Protein Playing Cards
(page 116). Color the pictures and cut apart the
cards.

Laminate the cards for durability.

Directions

1. Read one of the books about protein to the
   children. Explain that protein is important
   because it provides us with the nutrients
   that build muscles and bones and help us
   have energy. Lead the class in a discussion
   about what would happen to us if we didn't
   eat enough protein.

2. Next, lead the children in a discussion
   about healthy protein choices. Explain that
   chicken nuggets, although protein, are not
   the healthiest choice. Then teach the
   children the following song:

Powerful Protein
*(Sung to the tune of Head, Shoulders,
Knees and Toes)*

Chicken, turkey, pork, and beef!

Pork and beef!

Sausage, hot dogs, drumsticks, too!

Drumsticks, too!

Protein is what helps our bodies grow!

It's the fuel that makes us go!

Makes us go!

3. Finally, show the children the Protein
   Playing Cards. Have the children name the
   protein sources. Then have the children
   play concentration with the cards.

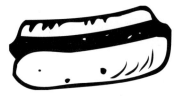

Protein Playing Cards

Make two copies of the cards below. Color, cut, and laminate to play.

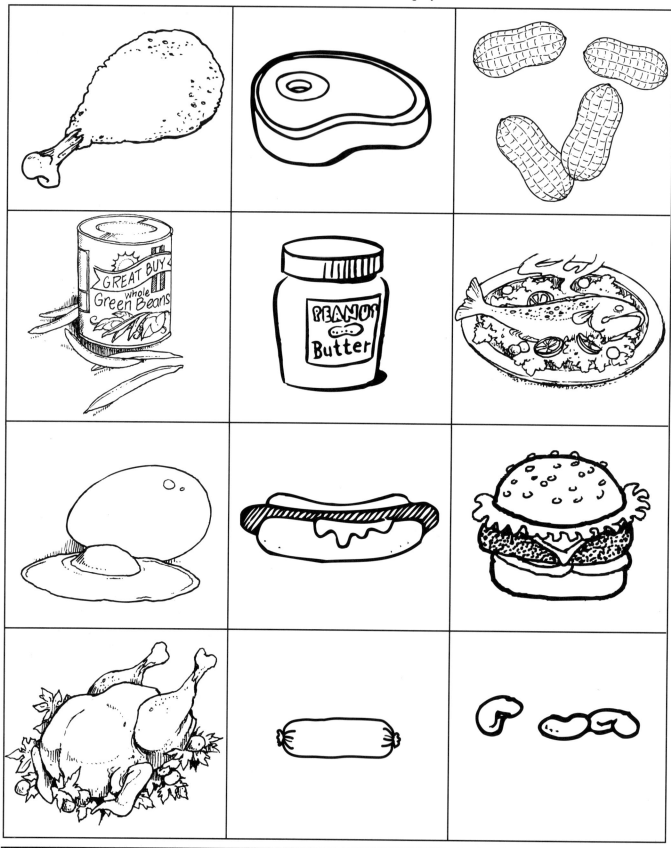

Makes 32 chicken nuggets.

Ingredients

$1\frac{3}{4}$ cups herb-seasoned crumb stuffing mix

$\frac{1}{4}$ cup grated Parmesan cheese

3 tablespoons margarine

$\frac{1}{4}$ cup low-fat buttermilk

$\frac{1}{4}$ teaspoon of ground black pepper

4 boneless, skinless chicken breasts
(approximately 1 pound)

Preparation done without the children

Rinse the chicken and pat dry. Cut chicken into 32 chunks of the same size. (Each chicken breast should give you 8 chunks or pieces.)

Directions

1. Preheat the oven to 450°F.

2. Put the stuffing mix into a resealable bag. Crush the crumbs by rolling and pressing the resealable bag. Add the parmesan cheese. Reseal the bag and shake it to mix the ingredients.

3. Melt the margarine. Place the margarine, buttermilk, and pepper in a shallow bowl. Stir the mixture.

4. The adult will dip each chicken chunk into buttermilk mixture, covering all sides, letting the extra buttermilk mixture drip off. Then the adult will place three dipped chunks at a time into bag of crumbs and seal bag tightly. The children can shake the bag until the chicken pieces are evenly coated with crumbs.

5. The adult will place coated nuggets on an ungreased baking sheet. Continue working in this manner until all of the chicken nuggets have been prepared.

6. Place baking sheet in the oven. Bake the nuggets for four minutes, then turn them over and continue baking for four to five minutes, or until the nuggets are a medium golden brown.

Serve nuggets immediately.

Note: Only adults should handle raw chicken. Wash hands regularly.

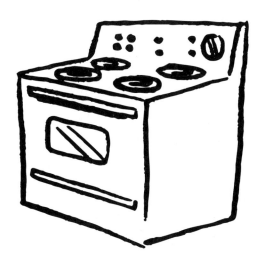

Recipe: Turkey and Stuffing Roll-Ups

This recipe makes 20 servings.

Ingredients

$\frac{1}{4}$ cup chicken broth

$1\frac{1}{4}$ teaspoons coarse ground black pepper

$1\frac{1}{4}$ teaspoon ground thyme

$1\frac{1}{2}$ cups celery, diced

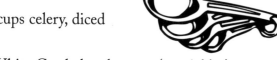

10 White Castle hamburgers (no pickles)

20 slices turkey luncheon meat

This recipe contains ingredients from the following food groups:

Meat and beans

Vegetables

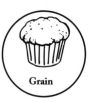
Grain

Directions

1. Preheat oven to 350°F.

2. Have the children help tear the defrosted White Castle hamburgers into pieces. Put these pieces in a large mixing bowl.

3. Add the diced celery and seasonings to the hamburger mix and toss well. Add the chicken broth and mix well.

4. Put the stuffing mix in a pan and cover it with aluminum foil.

5. Cook the stuffing at 350°F for 30 minutes.

6. When it is finished cooking, let cool to a temperature that can be handled by the children. Then give each child a piece of turkey.

7. Have each child spoon some of the stuffing mix on his or her turkey slice and then roll it up.

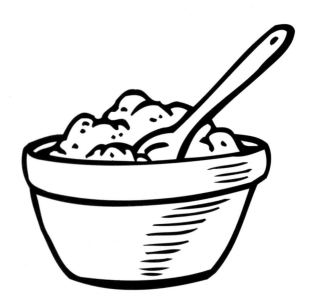

Eat and enjoy!

Skip, Skip, Skip to My Lou!

Demonstrate how to skip. Have the children practice skipping around the playground, to the cafeteria, to the bus or car line. Set up a simple obstacle course by arranging orange cones in a zigzag pattern and have the children skip through the pattern.

Walk a Straight Line

Demonstrate how to walk in a straight line, heel to toe. Then challenge the children to practice walking backward in a straight line, heel to toe! Have the children pretend to walk on a tightrope in this fashion too. Observe as the children walk this way. Do they need to have arms outstretched or can they walk this style with their arms at their sides?

Talent Show

Hold a talent show where the children can demonstrate their gross motor skills, exercise techniques, and flexibility one at a time. Praise all of the children for their talents and have the children cheer for their friends.

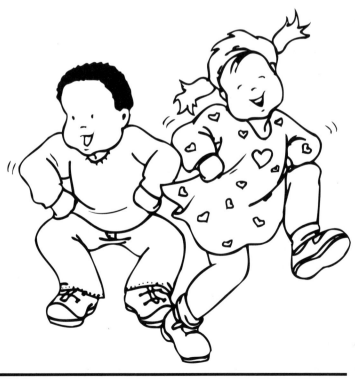

Many Meats Patterns

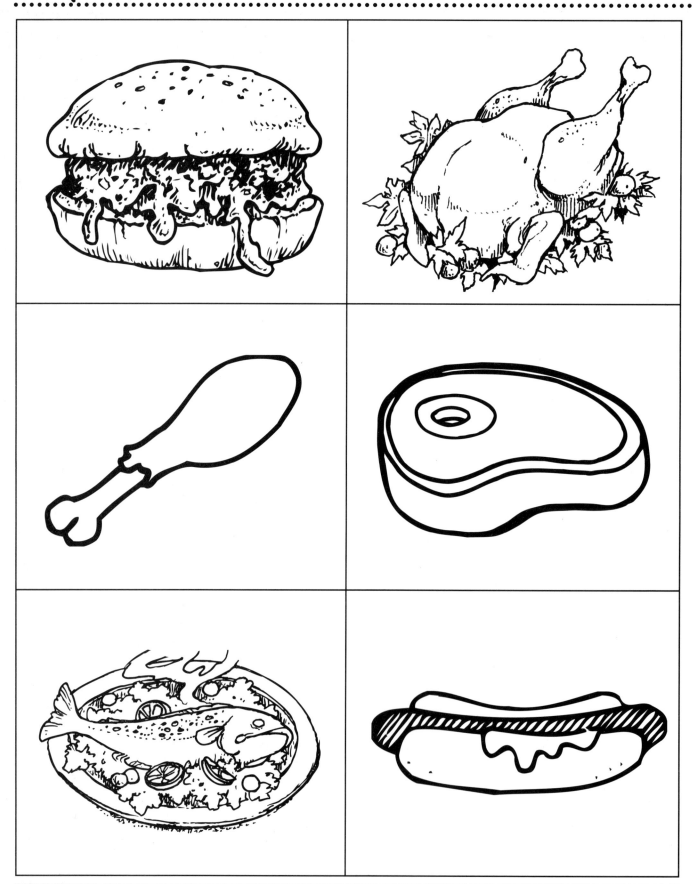

Lessons and Activities for Week Twenty-Three: TV Time Verses

Materials

Chart paper

Marker

The Berenstain Bears and Too Much TV by Stan and Jan Berenstain (Random House Books for Young Readers, 1984)

Lesson

1. Write "TV" on the board. Lead the class in a discussion about their favorite television shows. Write the names of their favorite shows on the board. When the children have named all of the shows they can think of, have them help you count how many they thought of.

2. Then write "play" on the board. Lead the class in a discussion about their favorite things to do that keep them moving. Have them name all of their favorite active activities (not playing video games, computer games). Write the children's favorite active activities on the board. Then have the children help you count how many they thought of.

3. Compare the two lists. Talk about which one had more suggestions. Ask the children if they think they spend more time watching television or playing. Have the children share their thoughts.

4. Then read *The Berenstain Bears and Too Much TV* to the children. Lead the class in a discussion about what happens to the Bear family when they are watching too much television. Have the children share their thoughts about what happened as a result of Mama Bear's decision to ban television for a week.

5. Ask the children how they would spend their time if they were not allowed to watch television. Discuss how the children would feel physically if they spent more time playing than sitting watching television. Suggest that next time they are watching television they should turn it off after one show and find something fun and active to do instead.

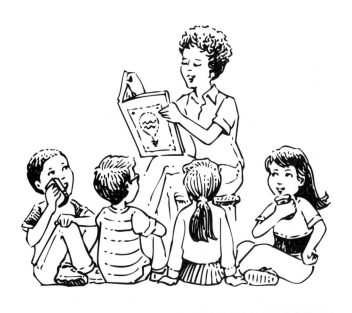

TV Time Verses Playtime Graph

Name _____

Date _____

Directions:

Keep track of how many hours you watch television this weekend. Keep track of how many hours you spend being active. Color in one box for each show. Color in one box for each game or activity.

Saturday

Sunday

This recipe makes 20 servings.

Ingredients

1 can chickpeas, drained

$\frac{1}{4}$ cup lemon juice (Use fresh if possible, the children can help you squeeze it.)

$\frac{1}{4}$ cup olive oil

1 clove garlic, crushed or minced

For dipping

Pita bread cut into small pieces

Baby carrots

Cucumber slices

Celery sticks

Broccoli spears

Red or yellow peppers, thinly sliced

Directions

Put all of the ingredients into a food processor and blend until smooth.

Serve with pita bread or cut up vegetables.

This recipe contains ingredients from the following food groups:

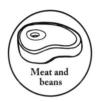
Meat and beans

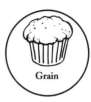
Grain

Fats, oils, and sweets

Exercises, Stretching, and Movement Activities

The children can increase their flexibility while forming their bodies into shapes that can be seen in nature. These stretches are influenced from traditional yoga poses.

The Mountain

For this stretch, the children will begin by standing with their feet shoulder length apart. They will bend at the waist and put their hands, fingers pointing forward, flat on the ground as far in front of them as necessary for them to be able to keep their knees straight. They should breathe in and out three times, slowly before standing up.

This is the "Downward Dog" yoga pose. It stretches the spine and hamstrings and increases flexibility.

Butterfly

For this stretch, the children will sit on the floor, with their knees bent and the soles of their feet touching. They will gently bounce their knees, trying to make them tap the floor five times. Repeat this three times.

This stretch strengthens lower back, groin, and hips.

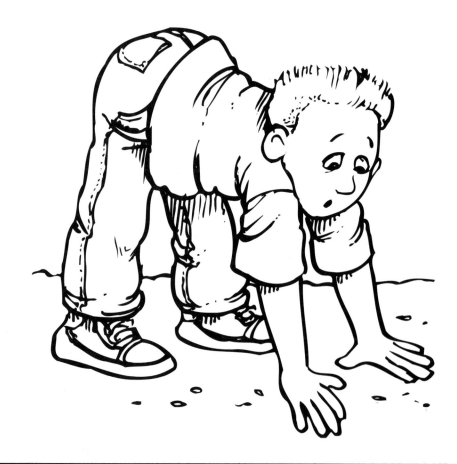

Directions:

Color in one punching glove for each serving of protein that you eat each day. Try to eat 5 ounces each day!

Monday	Tuesday	Wednesday	Thursday	Friday

What Do I Eat?

Keep track of what you eat for a whole day. Each time you eat something from the following food groups, color in one of the pictures in the column. Ask an adult to help you. See how close you are to eating the all of the foods that can help to keep you healthy.

Grains...6 a day

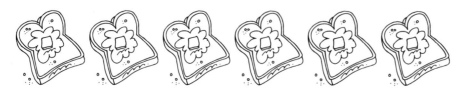

Vegetables...2 $\frac{1}{2}$ cups a day

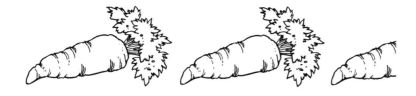

Fruits...1 $\frac{1}{2}$ cups a day

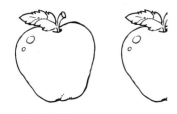

Milk...2 cups a day

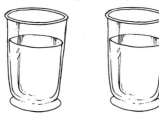

Meat and Beans...5 a day

Healthy Eating Rules

(Sung to the tune of If You're Happy and You Know It)

The food pyramid was made for us. (Yes, it was!)
The food pyramid was made for us. (Yes, it was!)
It shows us the way to eat healthy everyday.
The food pyramid was made for us. (Yes, it was!)

You'll have energy when you eat grains! (Whole grains, too!)
You'll have energy when you eat grains! (Whole grains, too!)
Cereal and bread and pasta are what it says.
You'll have energy when you eat grains! (Whole grains, too!)

Veggies have many colors and lots of crunch! (Try some soon!)
Veggies have many colors and lots of crunch! (Try some soon!)
Beans and salad, too, try them they're good for you!
Veggies have many colors and lots of crunch! (Try some soon!)

Fruits are sweet and juicy and good for you! (Yes, they are!)
Fruits are sweet and juicy and good for you! (Yes, they are!)
Bananas, apples and grapes, many colors, many shapes!
Fruits are sweet and juicy and good for you! (Yes, they are!)

Dairy is loved by kids everywhere! (2 cups a day!)
Dairy is loved by kids everywhere! (2 cups a day!)
Milk, yogurt, cheese, and ice cream if you please!
Dairy is loved by kids everywhere! (2 cups a day!)

Protein builds bones and muscles, too! (Makes us strong!)
Protein builds bones and muscles, too! (Makes us strong!)
Fish, meat and beans, you know just what I mean.
Protein builds bones and muscles, too! (Makes us strong!)

The food pyramid was made for us. (Yes, it was!)
The food pyramid was made for us. (Yes, it was!)
It shows us the way to eat healthy everyday.
The food pyramid was made for us. (Yes, it was!)

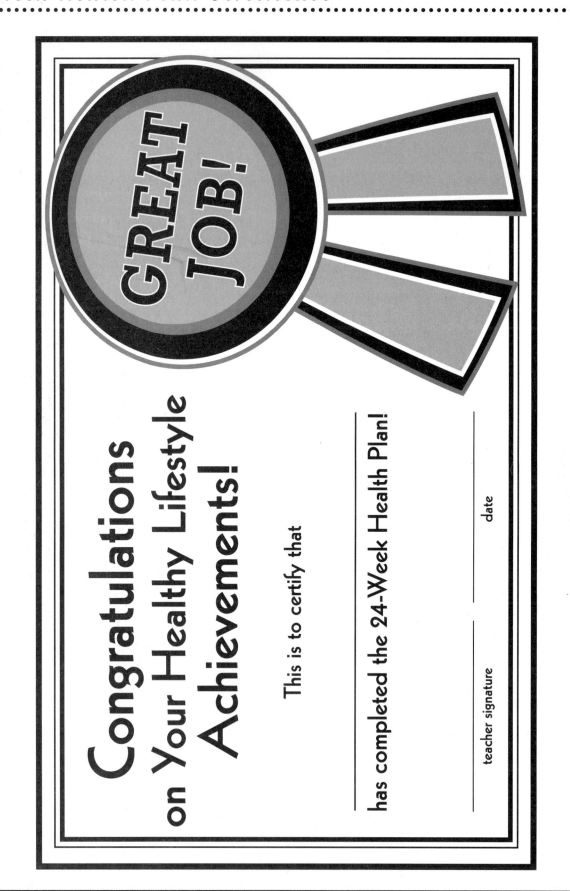

GREAT JOB!

Congratulations
on Your Healthy Lifestyle
Achievements!

This is to certify that

has completed the 24-Week Health Plan!

_____
teacher signature

_____
date

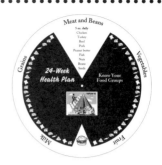

Cut out the circles and put together by pushing a brad through the center of the wheels. Rotate the top wheel to find information on the food groups. Turn the wheel over for activity ideas.

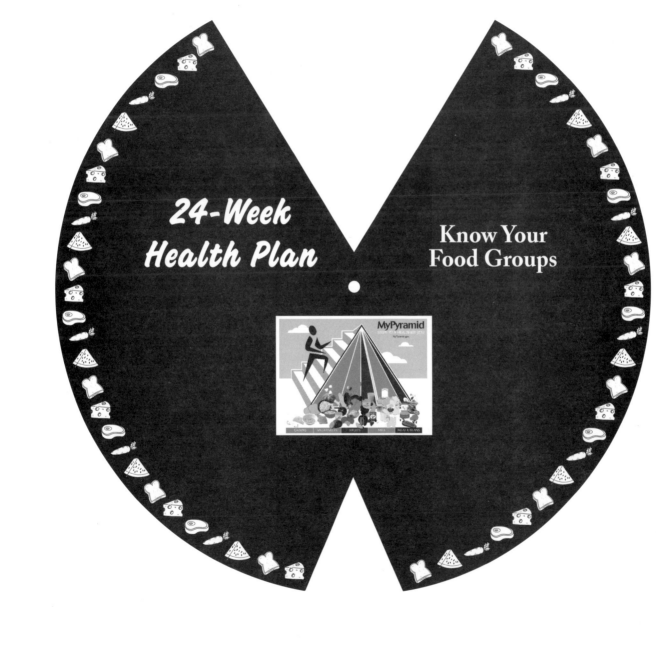

24-Week
Health Plan

Know Your
Food Groups

24-Week Health Plan

Gross Motor Milestones and Activity Ideas

3-Year-Olds

- Walk forward
- Walk backward
- Walk sideways
- Throw a ball
- Catch a ball
- Kick a ball forward
- Walk up stairs

4-Year-Olds

- Balance on one foot for 5 seconds
- Hop on one foot
- Catch a bouncing ball
- Pedal and steer a trike
- Turn a somersault
- Skip around an obstacle
- Climb up and down a slide

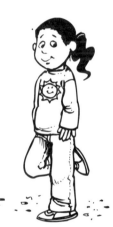

5-Year-Olds

- Run on tiptoes
- Walk on balance beam
- Jump rope
- Gallop
- Walk up and down stairs without a railing
- Move rhythmically to music
- Try complex coordination skills like dancing, swimming, ice skating

6-Year-Olds

- Play hopscotch
- Run skillfully
- Kick a ball accurately
- Jump over low items
- Hula hoop
- Walk forward heel-to-toe
- Hop on either foot 10 or more times

Published by Totline. Copyright protected.
1-57029-519-2   *24-Week Health Plan*

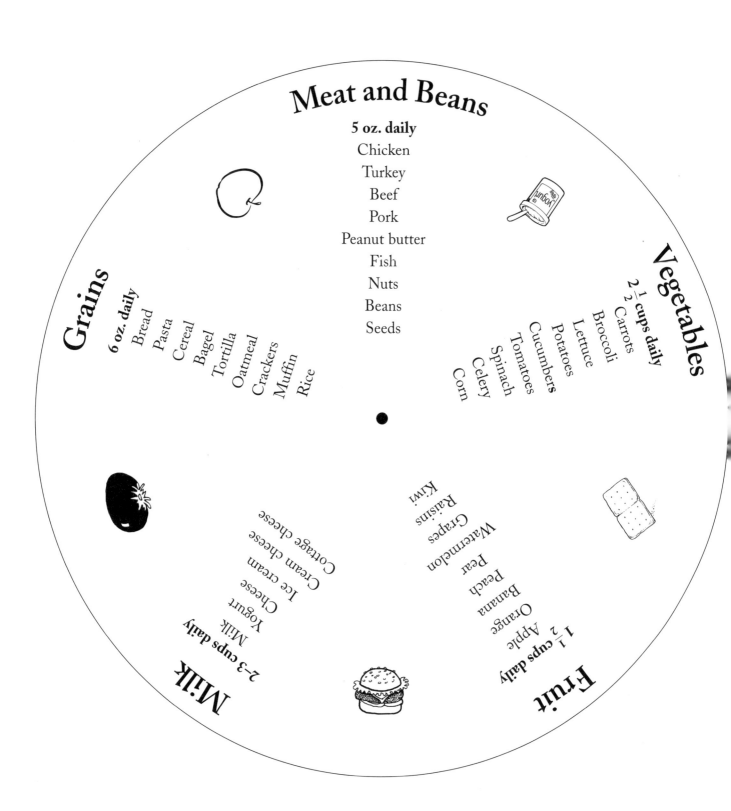

Meat and Beans

5 oz. daily

Chicken
Turkey
Beef
Pork
Peanut butter
Fish
Nuts
Beans
Seeds

Grains

6 oz. daily

Bread
Pasta
Cereal
Bagel
Tortilla
Oatmeal
Crackers
Muffin
Rice

Vegetables

2 ½ cups daily

Carrots
Broccoli
Lettuce
Potatoes
Cucumbers
Tomatoes
Spinach
Celery
Corn

Milk

2–3 cups daily

Milk
Yogurt
Cheese
Ice cream
Cream cheese
Cottage cheese

Fruit

1 ½ cups daily

Apple
Orange
Banana
Peach
Pear
Watermelon
Grapes
Raisins
Kiwi